Injury Prevention

Optimizing Performance Through Injury Prevention, pain-relief

(Essential Elements of Optimal Lifelong Fitness and Injury Prevention)

William Ruiz

Published By **Jackson Denver**

William Ruiz

All Rights Reserved

Injury Prevention: Optimizing Performance Through Injury Prevention, pain-relief (Essential Elements of Optimal Lifelong Fitness and Injury Prevention)

ISBN 978-1-77485-951-3

No part of this guidebook shall be reproduced in any form without permission in writing from the publisher except in the case of brief quotations embodied in critical articles or reviews.

Legal & Disclaimer

The information contained in this ebook is not designed to replace or take the place of any form of medicine or professional medical advice. The information in this ebook has been provided for educational & entertainment purposes only.

The information contained in this book has been compiled from sources deemed reliable, and it is accurate to the best of the Author's knowledge; however, the Author cannot guarantee its accuracy and validity and cannot be held liable for any errors or omissions. Changes are periodically made to this book. You must consult your doctor or get professional medical advice before using any of the suggested remedies, techniques, or information in this book.

Upon using the information contained in this book, you agree to hold harmless the Author from and against any damages, costs, and expenses, including any legal fees potentially resulting from the application of any of the information provided by this guide. This disclaimer applies to any damages or injury caused by the use and application, whether directly or indirectly, of any advice or information presented, whether for breach of contract, tort, negligence, personal injury, criminal intent, or under any other cause of action.

You agree to accept all risks of using the information presented inside this book. You need to consult a professional medical practitioner in order to ensure you are both able and healthy enough to participate in this program.

Table of contents

Chapter 1: Muscular Soreness 1

Chapter 2: Fatigue 18

Chapter 3: The Sleeping Habit................ 30

Chapter 4: Stress................................... 38

Chapter 5: Illness 45

Chapter 6: Load Monitoring................... 50

Chapter 1: Muscular soreness

A common topic in the health- and fitness industry is muscular soreness. There are many claims for remedies. In addition, there are many pro-tips and ideas to minimize the effects of this issue. A lot of evidence is not conclusive about the possible solutions. Contrastwater therapy is the preferred method. This is where an individual will spend an agreed amount of time (usually 1 min) in an ice-cold bath. The water temperature should be between 10 and 15 degrees Celsius. After that, they will be able to contrast their bodies and take a bath for 1 minute. They should rotate for between them for at least 5-7 minutes before switching to cold. This allows for temperatures to alternately constrict (cold) and open (hot). This is believed to reduce swelling and inflammation. In order to reduce muscle soreness, it is important to reduce the inflammation phase.

DOMS is thought be caused by muscle contractions that produce too much strain.

This causes cell membrane disruption of the structural protein in muscle. Repetitive muscular contraction triggers a low level of inflammation in the body. This could be due to a degree of microtrauma within the skeletal muscle. It is thought that this occurs 48-72 hours after exercise.

Clinically speaking, we notice a marked stiffness of soreness and tenderness when palpating. This tends to develop within the first 1-2 day, peaking around day 2 or 3. This tenderness to palpation typically disappears in 5-7 days. Passive stretching the muscle can aggravate the pain. DOMS can cause muscle weakness in the short-term. This has been shown to be associated with an increase in creatinekinase. Creatine kinase is an enzyme found within skeletal muscle tissue. When muscle damage is greater than normal, it can be detected in blood.

PRO-TIP #1: Different muscle contractions, different muscular damage

It is important for you to know that there are different types of muscle contractions. They have an impact on how severe cell swelling, inflammation, or muscular damage occurs at a physiological scale.

Some exercises, velocity rates and loading rates can have an impact on the severity of DOMS.

Exercising in eccentric ways, for instance, is thought to cause intracellular fibre swelling that can be associated with muscle soreness or stiffness.

This is an extremely valuable fact to have as it can greatly improve your exercise regimen and enable you to offer tailored training strategies to anyone at any stage of their training program. (Think about the viral Nordic Hamstring Curl that was shared on social media. People programmed them in three sets of 15 and then wondered if their hamstrings hurt for 2 weeks.

Qualifying and quantifying muscle soreness

It is important to keep track of the client's soreness when it comes to practical application. Not only should we monitor the soreness in terms of its severity, but also the muscle groups and specific body areas. Once you have started to track it (and we will discuss how to do this later in the book), you can start to make maps and predictability charts according to which body areas are becoming sore during which phases of the program. For example, you could map out which days in the week's plan, which week in the monthly load cycle, which exercises, sets, repetitions or weights. You get the idea. There are many ways to extrapolate this information. But the devil is always in the details. Each client's body reacts to exercise and stress differently. This is crucial to remember. Learn as much about your client's body and its responses as you would from your own. You should examine both the good and the negative. There will always be programming mistakes, but this isn't the most important thing. It is crucial that you understand the reason behind your programming mistakes so that your coaching abilities can be improved.

Case Study 1: Soreness

Client 1 begins to lift weights. They are instructed to deadlift the stiff-legged leg at 12 sets with a 4 seconds eccentric and a 1 second concentric repetition tempo. For four weeks, client 1 will use a weight 75% higher than their maximum repetitions per week. Regularly graded the client's hamstring soreness, and they have noticed an increase in their strength a few days later. The soreness will usually return to baseline in the second week. This would be a typical presentation to such a program.

After week 4, however, the client is complaining of stiff hamstrings and back pain. They are too stiff to even consider training in your session. This client wishes to get a week of rest before they return. They expect their back pain to be under control by that time. The muscular soreness charting you have taken shows that their hamstring soreness did not go back to baseline in weeks 3, 4 and 5. In fact, it was worse in those two weeks. It is possible to conclude that a review at Week 3 with alternate exercise or deloading would have helped to return the client to their baseline soreness and allowed them to continue with their sessions. You would get better results, less business loss and most importantly, more trust in your ability deliver what you say (your reputation and integrity). This will ensure your clients return to you again and again. By winning the battles that create future revenue streams, you can ensure your long-term success. A demonstrated ability to listen to clients will not only keep them comingback, but will also help generate word-of–mouth leads that will bring you new clients.

According to my experience, body charts detailing are the best method for monitoring soreness. A body chart detailing all major muscle groups can be used to create a simple Likert scale ranging from 1-5 up to 10 and ranging from the least severe pain to the most severe. I prefer the scale 1-10. It is what people are most familiar with and it is well conceptualized. Depending on whom you are training you will choose the muscle groups that you think would be most beneficial to your client. It's not a first date, or a job interview. Make it quick and efficient. You might be interested in the shoulders, pecs., triceps., forearms., stomach, abs., glutes., quads., hamstrings.

PRO-TIP #2, Upper and Lower Back Segments

Divide the back into two segments. Each segment will provide you with slightly different information. This can be used for cueing you to see which part of your client's programming may be working well. The thoracic spine, which is the upper back, is primarily involved in extension and rotation. This makes it easier to pinpoint what programming influences this area. This compares to the lumbar, which is more focused on remaining "neutral". I placed "neutral" in quotes marks because I don't believe there is neutral. There is no scientific neutral spine. There are two options: too much flexion which loads the tissues that restrain low-lumbar flexion (lumbar disk and supportive ligaments) and too little extension which increases the compression load on the tissues. (facet joint or supportive ligaments)

Refer to our soreness charting. Once you have gathered information about the severity, location, and duration of each session, it's time to ask your client what their soreness levels are. If you do this consistently, it will become almost automatic for your client and the process will be much faster. Your client will tell you, "How is your soreness today?" (often referring to last session). Simple, fast, effective. Take a look at the list and you'll be able to quickly review it and keep track.

Physiological Changes, Pain and Muscle Inhibition

I already discussed the physiological changes seen in DOMS patients. You will notice a decrease in muscle length. This can cause reduced joint range and motion, decreased strength and power output, tenderness, pain, and reduced muscle tension. Let's use the Case Study 1 client as an example. If they have severe muscular soreness it is possible to infer that their clinical markers show a decrease of at least 1, and possibly all of them. (We will come back to why severe pain is important later).

What is our knowledge regarding injury risk? DoMS is known to cause strength deficits, neurological inhibition, muscle weakness changes, decreased flexibility, decreased range of motion and neurological inhibition. Cause and effect. These factors affect the risk of injury and can push it to high or low. They also work in conjunction. These boxes must be checked more often to make the soft tissues or joints more susceptible to injury.

Let's explore the relationship of pain and muscle inhibition. It's a fact we all know that when something is painful, our instinct is to avoid the painful stimulus. Normal response is to stop doing it again. You keep the memories of that experience in your subconscious. It is the curator of experiences. It processes it and makes it unpleasant. It attaches the idea of a harmful, negative outcome to that experience, and then programs you to avoid such an experience in future. Over many years, our brains have been able to do this for millions of times. This is the key function of how we learn through experience: When an event occurs, we process all the information. This includes everything that our 5 senses see in the event environment. We also feel how the event made them feel. The information is processed and stored.

Take into account post-traumatic stress disorder, (PTSD). You might be familiar with the symptoms and how they relate to psychological triggers. This is your subconscious at its best. People are often afraid to drive or get in a vehicle again after being in car accidents. The brain associates the environment and actions with a perceived threat. The brain might replay an unpleasant experience if it detects a similar environment through the five senses in order to avoid it.

Muscular pain is governed by the nervous system. Without getting into details, a muscle contracture occurs when the brain releases neurotransmitters, which have a chemical interaction to the muscle cells, and fires off an electrical signal. When muscular microtrauma occurs (DOMS), the impulse is registered by the brain and the muscle contracts. Inflammatory markers also stimulate pain receptors, which are activated when there is muscular microtrauma. Simply put, muscle contraction is what causes pain. The brain doesn't just send messages; it also receives these messages. It learns from painful stimulus and associates pain with muscle contraction. This is similar to the nail in your foot scenario. It will attempt to avoid it by trying down-regulating motor neurons' excitability (neural inhibitor). This will result in a delayed contraction and reduced force development. It also means that peak strength values are lower. Thus, there is an increased risk of injury.

We've discussed resistance-based exercises, but what about more cardiovascular-intensive exercise? Experiences of severe DOMS may also negatively impact endurance events. We notice a decrease of economy and impaired glycogen repletion. Glycogen, which is the main fuel source for muscles during prolonged bouts aerobic exercise, must be restored after intense bouts. Another indicator that you are at risk of injury is muscle fatigue. (See Step 2). This is especially important for injury mitigation and performance in long-bout repetitive exercise forms.

The art vs. the science of coaching

Each step of this book can help you begin to collect the true value these screening tools. You will be able learn about your clients, find out who is more adept at training methods, and get concrete data on how you can manage client injuries. This is just one part of the 6-step algorithm that drives injury rates towards zero. For you this means zero missed sessions and no setbacks. Science also helps you determine how to maximize performance and deliver the best results for your clientele.

Our clients have shared their muscle soreness data with us and we have explained how this affects the muscular system. Furthermore, we can also take the records and extract the time it took to recover from an exercise session. Client 1 experienced recovery within 2 days following their exercise. This is if Client 1 was in the first two weeks. This is completely normal after doing heavy, eccentric exercises. Now, consider Client 2. They both perform the same exercise using identical parameters. However, they report soreness up to 4 day after training. Which client is most at risk from overtraining? Which client is at greater risk of injury

There are many reasons why certain people adapt faster than others. Some people recover faster. Some people change their body composition faster than others. Why is Usainbolt able to run the 100m faster than he can? Eliud Pipchoge is able to run a marathon in less than 2 hours, despite some controversy. Why are some football players able to play in all rounds while others have trouble with'soreness' season after season? Genetic expression can explain some of these differences. Another factor is the age. It is well known that older people recover quicker than younger individuals. It doesn't really matter why these differences exist. You must focus on who responds in which manner. This skill should be transferable and can be used by everyone who uses your services.

This is where you might wonder, "How severe is too much?" "What margin of risk?" Both these are valid questions, and they should be answered. You don't want to wrap your client up in bubble wrap. But, you also don't want your client to fail. This is where science meets the art and coaching. This is a skill that too many coaches and trainers have failed to master. Your ability to compete or maximize your client's goals, and your results for them, are all things that you need to master. The ideal scenario is one that balances push and recovery. This is discussed in Step 6, which focuses on managing the client's training load.

Now, it is crucial to not only determine how much the client reacts to an exercise stimulus, such as the intensity and muscle or body part affected, but also to determine their recovery times and rate, and, most importantly, any changes in their body reaction over time. Without proper analysis and intervention strategies, data are just marks. This will allow you to see the trend over time, which will enable you to identify the performance, injury, and overtraining peaks.

It is good to notice a reduction in soreness over time. This is what most trainers use. You can be among the top 1% in your industry if this is what you desire. Do you want to see less soreness? What about increases in your client's training metrics or KPIs (1RM), peak velocity, sprint times over a certain distance, peak height jump, jointROM, etc. No matter what your objective measure of performance gains, tracking them will show you how your push and recovery are working in your clients' favor. It doesn't mean you shouldn't take strength tests every few days, or do a 2km trial run each week. Analyzing should occur within the timeframes for physiological adaptation. The science and the arts merge when you create comparative data between your wellness screenings and your performance testing. Sometimes the reverse is true. A client may be tracking within their normal physiological expectation of muscular pain, but when performance testing results are available, you discover that they have lost some muscle soreness. Now, you know that your client has been lacking in training and could use some more guidance.

Sometimes you may not achieve the perfect balance and there will always been reasons. The more data that you analyse and track, the more you'll master the process. You will have the knowledge to determine when to drive clients or athletes, when it is best to substitute or back off, and when to encourage, modify, or re-assure. You have full control over the program, the outcome and how it is run.

Chapter 2: Fatigue

You must also take into account fatigue when assessing your client/athlete's performance, injury risk, or overall health. Fatigue comes as many forms. Each one can have a negative impact on the performance level required to stay injury-free or at low risk. The greatest failures of humanity have been caused by lapses of concentration, degrading sharpness, and a decrease in cognitive or bodily output due to success's dark passenger.

Fatigue management is an essential part of client success. However, it is not common to know how fatigue can affect the body physiologically.

The term mental or cognitive exhaustion refers to a psychobiological condition caused by prolonged periods or prolonged bouts of cognitively demanding activity. This could lead to an increase in risk or a greater likelihood of training errors. This can be manifested in client behavior or subjective reporting. The most obvious indicators are tiredness or feelings of fatigue, decreased energy, decreased motivation, or a decline of alertness. We recognize mental fatigue as decreased accuracy in physical movements, decreased time-to-epuion, reduced reaction time, and on a deeper basis, altered brain activity and neural synaptic functioning. When we take into account that mental fatigue can trigger these responses, we can see the effect it has on injury risk as well on client performance and achievement.

Injuries can result from alterations in accuracy or body position. In my career as a physiotherapist, I have seen a lot of injuries due to fatigue-induced movement error and body position. The body can become more tired at both the physical and neural levels. As a result, there is a tendency to make mistakes in movement. These errors can then cause abnormal or dangerous loading on the body's soft tissue.

Case Study 2 ACL Reflux

Fatigue-induced joints position error is one the main risk factors for ACL fracture. ACL ruptures happen in 70% of cases due to a noncontact incident. The common practice in comprehensive rehabilitation programs for sports injuries or musculoskeletal injuries is to treat the patient both at their normal cognitive state and as a complex cognitive demanding situation. Following is my process for rehabilitating a ACL injury. At first, an injured player may run at 60% their maximum speed and perform at approximately 45 degrees of their affected limb. This would be captured and slowed down to a fraction the original speed. A biomechanical analysis would follow to verify the correct body alignment, joint alignment, movement, and athletic technique. After this was achieved, there were gradual increases in cognitive demand. This is where things get more interesting. To illustrate, a player is given a ball as they move towards the cone. This increases cognitive tasking. The player has to track the ball, catch it and align their joints with the ball. This involves changing the body movement patterns, motor planning, and transferring the task from conscious to the effortless unconscious.

Once the basics are mastered, it's easy to move on. Mastery refers to the ability to move on slow-motion film in a way that is consistent with the previous. The same task might be completed under physical fatigue during the rehabilitation process. The athlete may be asked to run to fatigue and to continue the same exercise. Filming and analysis are done again and the execution of the move is analysed. The idea is for the athlete to become more familiar with what a match situation and demand might be. Sometimes, best practice can even be more aggressive that what is actually experienced during match play. This case is intended to show how damaging mental fatigue and an increase of physical body positioning can be. When you add in a decrease in time to fatigue, delayed reaction time, and a greater risk, your needle of risk moves to a higher level.

It seems that mental fatigue is only a problem with exercise that lasts for a long time. It is much more difficult to reach mental fatigue when there are very few tasks that require decision-making and cognitive tasking. Your clients may enjoy having all their training sessions written out for them. You might have several reasons for this, such as the fact that they don't know enough or lack the skills to do the task. But, they also have the option to prioritize and outsource their decision making efforts so they can put their energy and efforts into other tasks and sessions. Around 35,000 decisions are made each day. It is possible to reduce mental fatigue by taking fewer decisions. Steve Jobs was famous for his consistent use of the same black turtleneck, jeans, sneakers and sneakers each day. This allowed him to make more informed decisions on the most important matters. You can imagine a tank that is full. Your brainpower is what fills the tank. It is important to understand that each decision you make affects the amount of liquid in this tank. The impact your decision has on yourself and others directly correlates to the amount of liquid you have to withdraw.

But what about anaerobic, power or maximum strength exercises? These tasks (e.g. These tasks--e.g., performing 3 bench press reps and 3 broad jumps or participating in a 30 second sprint on the bike--are not as mentally challenging. The physical side effects of these exercises are more due to mental fatigue than to mental fatigue. These domains experience a decline due to a decrease in energy usage and a reduction in efficiency in the body's metabolic processes. Case Study 2: Recall our ACL client. This client was tested in cognitive tasking, as well physical fatigue scenarios, to help complete their rehab. We must also be aware of how fatigue can increase injury risk. We discussed in the previous chapters how muscular injury and changes in metabolism affect the body's ability to replenish glycogen stores. Because glycogen is the source of energy that allows muscular contractions to take place, it is obvious that maximal performance can be affected. In other words, injury susceptibility increases when there is insufficient muscular performance in relation strength and muscle power. This is especially true for those who notice a decrease of time to exhaustion. This means that fatigue, in any form, should be measured and quantified.

How to measure fatigue

I'm going to share with you the best and most effective methods that can be used to monitor client fatigue levels. Professional sport has long accepted the use of fatigue monitoring questionnaires. A majority of professional teams will monitor their athletes' fatigue status two to three times per week. The data is kept in a log and compared with training load exposures. These should be used as a guideline. This is very similar in concept to the Likert-scale for muscular soreness. This is an easy way to keep track of data. This will give you an idea of how your client might feel on the surface. It is a good way to see if physical fatigue and mental fatigue are caused by any of the biopsychosocial variables.

Measuring the heart rate

The autonomic nervous is closely associated with fatigue status. It is easy to determine if it works properly. Many people today have easy access to tools and gadgets that can measure heart rate. Training watches, and other devices for training, can now measure heart rate variability accurately. It is common knowledge that a drop in resting heart rates indicates an increase of cardiovascular fitness. It is an indicator of a positive body state that indicates the client or athlete is adapting well to the training stimuli they are receiving. This is easy and straightforward to track. Being aware of this is essential for your client's wellness. Once again, by analysing the trend, coaching your client will become easier. Your programming should not be able to detect an increasing trend. If you know that your client's resting pulse rate would be 60bpm but after a three-week training block, it registers 80bpm, this is an indication that they have been overtrained and need to be intervened.

Variability of heart rate

A second method that is used by elite athletes and many coaches in their training is the heart rate variability (HRV). It is another useful method to assess the fatigue status for your client or athlete. HRV refers the time that elapses between heart beats. We may think that our heart beats 60 times per second and therefore that we are able to hear every beat, but in reality, the rhythms of our hearts vary. For a healthy individual, the interval between two beats may be as short as 1.2 seconds and as long at 0.8 seconds. This variability is typical of a healthy autonomic nerve system and a body that's ready for loading. Thus, the more variable your heart rate is, the more prepared and adaptable you are. A decrease in HRV can indicate that the individual is being overtrained through fatigue and may be at risk of injury. Newer watches are able to calculate heart rate variability. This allows for easier monitoring both for the coach and the client. It reports the current heart rate, and graphs it over time. It is important to train your client in how to monitor it, and you can also monitor it on your behalf. This will ensure that you are successful at fatigue monitoring.

The same applies to fatigue data monitoring as it can for muscular soreness. This is how you can effectively manage your client's risk of injury, performance decrease, and overtraining. You can see signs that your client is beginning to overtrain, such as a decrease in heart beat variability or an increase at rest. This method of assessing fatigue status is the most reliable and effective. It uses objective data that is completely impartial, which gives accurate and reliable results every time. It takes out the personality who reports they are not fatigued, feel well, and aren't tired so they can keep going with every session. This can be a positive trait that you love coaching and a way to help your clients. If your body is not ready or in the best shape to work hard, it will not be able to give you a positive workout. Top-grade teams of athletes will recognize that athletes feeling tired, fatigued and worn down can be enough reason to decrease training load, substitute a gym session with a recovery session, or reduce field training time or intensity. This should make it easy for you consider how much you should push your client each week.

You must remember the art of coaching and the balance. Know when you should push your athlete. Overreaching and repetitive stress can often lead to the greatest gains. This is a tool that will help you identify what your clients are able to tolerate and what they can respond maximally to. Push them. Monitor their fatigue signs. Use it as a blueprint. Motivation is a powerful tool to combat mental fatigue. Low mental fatigue doesn't necessarily mean lower physical performance. Just think about the clients that you have had to train that just when they thought they wouldn't be able to complete that last rep, sprint, or burpee, thanks to positive talk or high energy verbal communication, they are able get over it. Mental fatigue gives the client the impression that they are working harder than their actual abilities. They have a different perception. Do not think that a corporate worker cannot work because they are tired from long hours. Measure, train, remeasure, analyse, and adapt. That's the secret principle.

Chapter 3: The Sleeping Habit

Step 3 is the most crucial pillar in the wellness screen. It can be a gateway to success or hinderance to performance. This pillar appears to have the ability to catch the flow-on effects one might experience from fatigue, muscle soreness, stress, illness, and more. Its ability to influence injury and poor performance is why it is so powerful.

This topic is constantly under investigation and many theories are being put forth about why sleep is important. Most believe that sleep refers to a period when the mind and bodies shut down and enter a rest phase. This is incorrect, however. The brain's active period of sleep is one that involves significant processing, strengthening and restoration. The exact mechanism of how our bodies get to sleep for extended periods of time and the reasons behind it is still unknown. The importance of sleep is much more significant than we originally thought. Millions of years worth of evolution did not make us who we are without a greater purpose. However, we are able to recognize some of the important functions of sleep. We all know that sleep is essential for our learning and development. It also helps us to retain and consolidate the memories we have from our daily activities in the morning. The brain processes quite a bit during sleep. It processes a lot of information, I really mean that. The majority of this is managed by our subconscious, or incognito brain. Overnight, little bits of information can be transferred from our shorter-term memory to our longer-term memory. It is also believed that the ability to sleep improves learning speed and skill acquisition.

Anecdotes are plentiful that illustrate how this happens. Personally, I experienced this first with music and my ability of playing the guitar. There were times when I could not nail a particular sequence or lick after hours of practicing. I would practice, record myself, then listen and it would never happen. The next time that I picked up an instrument, my first attempt would string together just like the stars aligned. It was as if the path had been paved. I was initially unsure why this happened. It makes complete sense now, that I am more conversant in the area. Overnight my brain would replay the exact sequence of musical notes, and I would begin to develop the fine motor skills necessary for me to match the music in my head.

This kind of learning and developing has been documented throughout the ages. Albert Einstein used routinely to sleep for 10 hour a night and took power naps throughout his day. He believed it made his brain work better and went on to do some incredible things.

It is clear that our sleep functions are to restore, rebuild, build muscle, repair tissues, and synthesizehormones. It is important to get enough quality sleep. We need it to be able to pay the taxes that training and life on the mortal coil take away from us. There is no such thing a "thing for nothing".

Even though your clients may believe sleep is only for the weak, they could be extremely talented and think that it is. However, this attitude is detrimental to injury risk reduction and performance. We see an increase in muscle damage, intramuscular inflammation/swelling, metabolic stress and hormonal changes after training efforts to achieve a fitness gain. Additionally, stress and fatigue can build up. All of these factors must be managed to restore the body's peak functioning order. If taken the proper steps, the body is capable of doing this feat well. Lack of sleep quality and quantity will cause your client to be more susceptible to injury and limit their ability for them achieve their goals.

Growth hormone, also known as peptide hormone, is released by pituitary. It is a wonderhormone in the body and was once called the "fountains of youth". Human Growth Hormone (HGH), is crucial in the regeneration of tissue, recovery from injury and fatigue, and skeletal development. This hormone is thought to improve the recovery rate from injuries, exercise, and even reduce the effects on ageing. It's interesting that the majority of HGH released is as a result either of exercise stimulation or during sleep. Journals have reported that as much as 75% of HGH is released during sleep. The amount of HGH released depends on age. It becomes most concentrated around the age of 30 and then slowly decreases. To ensure proper recovery from fatigue, muscle damage and hormonal secretions, the body needs to sleep.

Inadequate sleeping habits can also be detrimental to one's cardiovascular health. Research has shown how detrimental sleep deprivation is to one's fitness. We know that the aerobic energy system can suffer from a lack of 6 hours sleep. An individual's risk of injury increases if they have an increased level of fatigability, and a shorter time to exhaustion.

Quality of sleep measured and tracked

It is easy to measure and track soreness, fatigue, or both. All it takes is a simple client check in on a numerical scale between 1-10. The true meaning of this is the functional interplay between each pillar. Sleep has the deepest roots in all of the pillars, and is almost the puppet master that controls them all.

Case Study 3 The power and importance of sleep

Early on in my career, it was possible for me to see the impact sleep plays on rehabilitation and recovery. This was during my time as a private-practice clinician. My client was a Pacific islander man who loved his football. He was recovering from a serious work-related injury that had left him unemployed for more than 12 years. His symptoms were neck stiffness and weakness in the upper extremities. He also had numbness down his arms that he could not control. He was also unable to sleep for more than 1-2 hours per night. In addition to the physical limitations, this client also had to deal with psychosocial factors. This can have a wicked way of changing even the most brilliant personalities. The client was seen by a variety of specialists, including psychologists, therapists, and physical therapy. Only after the collaboration helped improve the client's sleep, his number rose from 1-2 to 6-7 hours. In just a few days all signs of muscular weakness, numbness, and muscle weakness were gone. His strength and ability to train in the gym was dramatically improved. As you can see, his mood also improved. Six weeks later, the client was successful in his work integration. I had a debriefing with the specialist that day and he stated strongly that sleep is the only thing that helped the client recover. This was the reason I decided to present this pillar. It has earned its place.

High quality sleep appears to be proportional to the other wellness tests. Clients who have a good quality sleep will report a lower rate of fatigue, sickness, soreness, and stress. This is also true for the opposite. Low quality sleep and lower numerical ratings will result in rises across all pillars. You need to be able to spot patterns in your clients' wellness and their reports across the board. This will allow you to be more targeted with your lifestyle and wellness coaching. This is how you can set yourself apart among the other average coaches. This will come from your ability and willingness to dig deeper and find out what is causing their overall wellbeing. All of this combined will ensure that you don't throw out the baby with all the other fish. This allows you to control your programming and eliminate the dangers of injury and overtraining. You should be systematic in your approach. You can't be deceived by numbers; they are your keys to success.

Chapter 4: Stress

Performance reduction and injury risk can be greatly reduced by reducing stress and responding to stress. Research into training was dominated in the past by focusing on the factors that would make an individual more susceptible to injury. You can see that psychosocial behavioural variables are becoming more prominent in the research. I believe that this is directly related to modern-day life. We are constantly under stress regarding our work and relationship statuses as well as financial and debt status. The negative effects of social media on self-image and how it can negatively impact our self-image are just some of the modern-day burdens.

Based on scientific evidence, it is clear that injury risk increases when there are too many stressors in our lives, such as somatic trait anxiety and ineffective stress-coping mechanisms. These risk factors include adverse life events and past injuries. This can result in a psychophysically maladaptive state.

This will lead to a problem state for your client if you fail to control these stressors.

In stressful situations, people can experience reduced attention, increased distraction, and more muscle-tendon tension. These are all factors that increase the risk of injury. Consider a time when you were unprepared, not resourceful, or lacking the skill set to accomplish a task in a stressful time. You might experience feelings of overwhelm, racing mind, uncontrollable thoughts, or tight muscles. You should not feel this way.

Trauma risk and psychosocial behavioural issues

It is becoming more common for psychosocial behavioural problems to be associated with higher injury risk. It is essential to assess the type of personality of an individual and how it may affect how they react to training stimulus. Also, where they rank on the injury-risk scale. Let's keep it simple. We can categorise people into optimists or pessimists to examine their responses to stress and the effects of injury. Pessimists tend to have more difficulty dealing with stress than optimists. Optimists are positively associated with emotional control. They can be proactive and deal with problems when they arise. True optimists tend to have poor coping skills and emotional distress. However, those with low optimism and life stress tend to be less effective at coping and react more slowly. It is also found that they have a faster recovery time after being actually hurt.

This is where wellness coaching pays huge dividends. A big advantage is the ability to actively identify, recognise and categorise client personality traits. This is a critical step towards understanding how you can keep clients healthy and moving forward. Social support and education about coping skills and strategies can positively influence the relationship between injury, stress, and social support. People with higher self confidence are more optimistic and have higher self esteem. They also tend to be more resilient than those who have lower self esteem. This makes them better able and more prepared to deal with life stresses, reduce injury risk, and speed up recovery between training sessions.

PRO-TIP #3, Meditation

This technique has been used by many of my clients to help with stress reduction and muscle tension. Simple meditation can make all of the difference. It is clear that we are all feeling more stressed these days. You can manage stress by focusing on positive emotions and releasing tension. Here's how. Close your eyes for at least one minute. Do a few extra deep breaths. Take 5 seconds inhale and 10 seconds exhale. After several rounds of this, scan the body. Recognize any areas that feel tight or tense. It is possible to shine a light onto the problem area, and it will be released. You should scan from head to tip, including the jaw and neck, shoulders and chest, as well as the diaphragm. This works well to reduce tension in the body. This trick I discovered after taking a freediving course.

The main idea behind freediving involves relaxing your muscles as much possible. The longer you can hold your breathe, the less oxygen you need. Relaxing your muscles can reduce your body's demand of oxygen, which will decrease your need for air.

It is essential to stress-free performance and getting the best from your clients. This is the job for which they will hopefully pay you. Stress should be seen as a sign from your body that you are preparing for something. It creates a state of high arousal that is vital for performance. Insufficient stimulation for something can lead to poor mental and physical preparation. This can hinder performance, making it impossible for you to reach your goals. A state of excessive arousal may also affect performance. Arousal in excess can lead to increased muscular tension and poor decision making. It can also cause a reduction in concentration and disruption of coordination. These are not all the ingredients necessary to make a PB.

Stress has physical side effects

It is hard not to notice the changes in hormone regulation and chemical alterations in the body. Cortisol has been called "the stress hormone". While the relationship between exercise and cortisol is complicated, it's clear that there is an increase in cortisol after any exercise. The intensity and duration of exercise, training experience and time of day all influence the degree of cortisol levels. Cortisol can be a positive response to psychological and physical stress. It aids the body to supply energy to its working muscles. But, cortisol levels can become a problem over time. This could occur due to high training volumes, poor recovery times, life stressors, and insufficient coping strategies. Catabolic hormones can cause muscle loss and damage, which can negatively impact exercise performance and muscle recovery. You will recall from the beginning of this book that muscle damage and decreased ability to recover increases injury risk. Cortisol is also known to suppress the immune response.

Cortisol can make you more susceptible to illness in the long-term, as discussed in Step 5.

Monitoring your client's stress levels is a smart idea. It is essential to monitor and analyze these changes for injury mitigation. It is vital to understand where your client is experiencing stress so that you can manage their injury risk. You can break it down into different sub-categories, such as general stress, stress from social situations, or feelings of pressure. All of these elements have an impact on one's level of stress. It is possible to pinpoint the area that is problematic and help you manage your client. Do you remember how optimism, self-efficacy and self-confidence are powerful predictors in injury risk? Asking about the client's feelings of achievement and optimism is a great way to learn more about their mental state.

Chapter 5: Illness

We briefly addressed illness in the previous chapter. It was recognized that illness can increase an individual's vulnerability to injury. We will use the term "illness" to refer to a compromised immune response. It is important to remember that exercise increases cortisol production and long-term, high-level exposure can lead to a debilitating effect on the body's immune systems. For cardiovascular training, higher intensities and longer durations of exercise (>60min) release significantly more cortisol that moderate or low-grade. It is catabolic in its nature and begins to degrade the body's capacity to repair or recover. This is a slow and gradual process that leads to a negative balance. To aid in physiological healing, long-term elevated levels continue to activate the immune system and create pro-inflammatory responses. This affects the immune system's ability to fight various pathogens, bacteria, and daily exposures to different microbes. This makes the body vulnerable to chronic fatigue and overtraining syndrome as well as a reduced ability to recover.

This is how it will impact your clients. It's just an outcome of all that we have discussed so far. Fatigue, impaired recovery (muscular injury), and increased stress levels can all contribute to an increase in injury risk. This shows how interconnected each of the pillars is and how they impact one another. It is an ever-changing, fluid situation. Although one pillar may be the most important, it is certain to have an effect on all others. Let's recall the analogy where these five pillars are responsible for supporting the roof of a church. If one pillar fails, the temple will be structurally compromised. Further stress is placed on other pillars.

How to monitor immunity

Now, unless your client has permission to give you blood samples each week, and you have access and the resources to do so, you may be wondering how you can screen them and map their immune system. It is impossible to pinpoint the exact immunity of a person using invasive methods. However, it is possible for a method to map the loading process. This method evaluates the current state of fatigue and their acquired fitness. Knowing that accumulated fatigue has a negative impact on the immune systems, it can be used to help you determine their current state. Apart from mapping your client's fatigue against their fitness level, you can also draw measures of their fatigue to determine what their physical state is.

A comparison between a fitness and fatigue function can help you to determine the athlete's performance. The direct relationship between training-performance and dose-response is directly proportional. Simply put, the greater your training, the better you perform. It is important to provide the right amount of training stimulus, at the right duration, frequency and intensity, in order to maximize your performance and minimize potential side effects such as fatigue, illness, injury and overtraining. Finding the perfect balance is an individual matter. It's highly dependent on both external and internal stressors.

Research is abundant on the impact of training volume and intensity on performance. It has been shown that performance increases with increased workload. Higher training intensity is associated with positive effects. Unfortunately, exercise training has a higher incidence of negative adaptations. The highest workloads are the most vulnerable to injury. You get more injured the harder you train.

This might be frustrating for those who are in the business and need to deliver results for their clients. Don't worry. Next chapter I will demonstrate how you can track and graph your clients' state of fatigue and their fitness. This will provide you with a graphic representation of your client's fitness level and their fatigue levels. The more fit an individual, the less susceptible they will be to injury. This is a battle-tested process that has been widely used in elite sporting and human performance settings.

You're done with the 5 wellness monitoring steps. Now it's time to move to step 6. This is what ties it all together and solidifies our 6-figure protection approach. This is the basis of all injury vs. Performance programming.

Chapter 6: Load monitoring

Here is my trade secret. It is still not available for commercial training. This method has been proven and tested at the highest level. The sixth step will give your sixth sense for predicting injury. It will help to establish risk mitigation and system systems before it's too much. This is the best way to keep multi-millionaire athletes from getting infected and unable to work for weeks or months. This ability is what sporting organizations pay millions for because every game missed by a star athlete equals millions of lost dollars. The same holds true for you and your clients. Each missed session is a financial cost and an opportunity lost to deliver what you promised: results.

Condition of fatigue, and state of health

It all boils down to load monitoring. That is, measuring fatigue and fitness. Let's start by defining these two terms. A state called fatigue is the exact condition your client will be in during their last week training. This will also be known as the acute workload. It's the total load that an individual has accumulated in the last week of training. An individual's fitness level is determined by the amount of training load they have accumulated in the previous month. This means that all of their training stresses are added together. This will allow you to determine their current level of fitness. You could, for example, say your client has been consistent with their training and hasn't missed one session. This would indicate that their current level of fitness is greater than if they had missed 20%.

Client success is negatively affected when injuries are common during physically-demanding tasks. We now know the secret to decreasing injury risk. The key is to find the workload that maximizes fitness and performance while minimizing injury risks. Here's the deal. To determine injury risk, you will need to compare your client's training state (fatigue) with the training loads that the athlete has been trained for (the state they are in the last 4 weeks). This allows the client to know if their ability to tolerate the training stimulus is greater or less than the acute workload.

PRO TIP 4: The fatigue to fitness ratio

This ratio will give you an indication of your client's loading status as well as their injury risk. The risk is greater if this ratio is high. Recalling high school math, in order to get the best results for your clients you must be able balancing the highest acute workloads, (injury protector adaptations), and the highest chronic workloads or fitness status. This will increase the ratio to a better number. A HIGHER CHRONIC WORKLOAD PROTECTS AGAINST INJURY WHEN THE ACUTE LOADING IS SIMILAR TO THAT OF THE CHRONIC WORKLOAD.

It is hard to balance science and art. It is also very individual. Each person reacts to loading in a different way. It is therefore impossible to create a general rule about what a safe load ratio should be. I have found that increasing the client's acute loading by more than 2-fold the fitness level increases the chance of injury. This is particularly true if it continues for two weeks. It is possible to observe a curious phenomenon with clients who are overloaded. It is common to see a delay between high loading and injury. Consider a client who was loaded at 2.5 times per week for two consecutive weeks. In the two weeks of high-load training, there is a good chance that you will not sustain an injury. Normally, injury occurs 2 weeks after the appropriate load increase. It is crucial to monitor this ratio every week and adjust as needed based on what load monitoring shows.

Arbitrary units are the best way to track workload. Take the RPE (rates perceived exertion from 0-10) immediately from the client once they have finished their session. Next, multiply this number by the length of the session.

Case Study 4: Tracking Workload

If your client reports a RPE value of 7 for a 60 minute session, their arbitrary work load is:

7 x 60 =420 units

If they had done this session three times during the week, and reported the same RPE every time, then their acute workload might be:

420 x 3, = 1260 units

The fatigue:fitness rate is the number of arbitrary units that you use for each session. The number of units you have completed in a given week of training determines your state of exhaustion. It is the summation of all training sessions during the week that determines the fatigue number.

This can be extended by taking the last 4 weeks of fatigue units and adding them together to calculate the average. Then we can determine the client's current fitness level and chronic workload. As an example, suppose that the 4-week average is 1000 units. This ratio is then:

1260:1000 = 1.26

When we take into account that more than 2 is injury risking loading, it can lead to a better physiological performance outcome. As a rule, below a ratio 1 will result in a loss of performance or fitness. Let's say you take the same client twice. They both have the same fitness level (1000). For the acute week, they train to a total of 775 units. This would result in:

750:1000 = 0.75

They need to be able to sustain or improve their fitness with the help of this training stimulus. You should also consider the client's training schedule and frequency. Tapering, de-loading, and other training methods may be appropriate for the client. It is up to each case.

My bonus material on bydesignbc.com.au contains more information on this method of visual analysis. Here's a table format demonstration that you can use to help your clients with their unique training needs and characteristics.

This method provides a reliable and quantifiable way to measure your client's loading. This will give you valuable insight into their injury risks and susceptibility. Clients with high levels of training will be more resistant to injury and have higher chronic loads. This doesn't mean your clients can't load harder or more frequently; it's just a way for you to gain insight into their current fitness levels and injury risk. There are clients that appear to be bulletproof. They will not give up no matter how heavy or complicated the load. These are your copers', and they can naturally load to higher extremes. Some clients may not even want to see a list of weights and their breakdown. Understanding your clients and how they react to stress is key to their well-being and the success of their work.

The 6 steps

Each of the six steps in the protection plan work together. They all work together and provide critical information. When administered correctly, your client should be able, at any moment, to classify their injury risk, performance level, and damage resistance. Before loading is determined, it's important to think about all pillars. Each stage should be carefully considered. There will be occasions when the loading of a client is perfect but one of their other pillars is flagging. This is just as dangerous as a 3.0 load ratio. You need to remember that each of these pillars are interconnected and all work together to promote the well-being of your clients. If you can master these pillars, you will be able to correctly load clients in all situations.

Strains or sprains to the ankle

You are more likely to sustain an ankle injury if you walk, jog and run. Ankle strains are the most common orthopaedic condition. These are a common injury and can happen at any age. Most likely, ankle sprains won't require special medical treatment. Knowing how to best manage the injury is a great help. It is possible to reduce pain levels, return faster to activities, save money on rehab bills, and prevent future injury.

The Journal of Sports Medicine (January 14, 2014) performed a meta-analysis of ankle sprains. It was found that women are at greater risk for ankle sprains than were men and that children are more likely than adults to injure their ankles. Indoor and court-based sports were the most risky. An ankle sprain may be caused by accidentally stepping on or slipping off your bed.

A sprain and strain are often both possible in an ankle injury. A ligament injury known as a sprain can be described as a strain. Ligaments connect bones to bone. Strains are injuries of muscles or tendons. A majority of cases involving an ankle injury will indicate that there was an injury both to a ligament or muscle. The treatment process is almost identical, regardless of whether there has been a strain or a sprain.

An ankle sprain happens when your ankle twists too far. The ligaments supporting the ankle are stretched or torn by this twist. A sprain could take anywhere from weeks to months to heal depending on the severity of the injury. The severity of an injury can be determined by how much pain you feel and how much swelling you have. This could indicate a longer recovery.

If the injury isn't treated properly, a chronically injured or severely sprained ankle could indicate ligament deficiencies. This could indicate that one or more ligaments in the ankle have been damaged or are significantly stretched. In these cases, an individual can learn to use motor control and muscle strength to manage pain and discomfort. Sometimes, surgery is required to repair torn or damaged ligaments.

You must receive proper treatment to ensure your complete recovery from your injury. Without proper treatment, you could sustain another injury. After you have suffered an ankle sprain, you are much more likely to sustain another.

There are many possible types of ankle sprains. However, the most common type is the lateral one. Initially, the lateral leg sprain will cause the foot to roll inward (or invert) further than normal. This causes a "sprain," or a strain of the lateral ligaments. It could also cause strains to the tendons and lateral muscles of the ankle. Peroneals are the muscles most often affected. In more severe cases the fibula bone, fifth metatarsal bone close to the pinky nail could also be broken or the tendon could burst from the bone.

Ankle Sprains

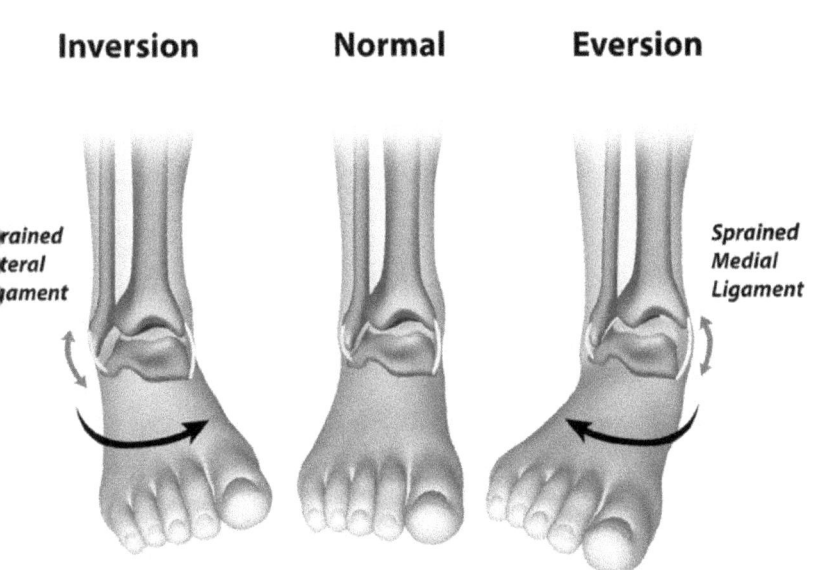

Medial sprains are caused by the foot rolling too far outward, or into eversion. This type of injury is to the inside portion the ankle. This type of injury occurs in contact sports. This happens when a contact sport player presses one's leg inward, causing a relative outward move onto the ankle. This motion is often blocked by the fibula. Fibular fractures are often associated with a sprain.

Another type is the syndesmosis, or high ankle injury. The syndesmosis is the fascia or ligamentous tissue that binds the tibia to the fibular. This type sprain accounts approximately 15% for all ankle sprains. This type is most common in American football and collision sports. Typically, the foot is rotated outside (outwardly) when there is a collision. This causes injury to the tissue between the bones. An additional mechanism that causes injury is when the feet are too bent up. This causes the bones of the foot to splay outwardly.

Many of this rehabilitation guide's treatment options are designed to treat lateral ankle injuries. But, the majority of the treatment advice can also be applied to any kind of ankle strain or sprain. The same treatment can be used for a Fibular Fracture, which may include surgical fixation of injuries, or any other foot/ankle injury. One must also consider possible weight bearing issues and wound treatment that might be required in the event of surgical intervention. You will need to note any special considerations or treatment advice for a certain type of injury.

Grading Ankle Strains or Sprains

SPRAINS

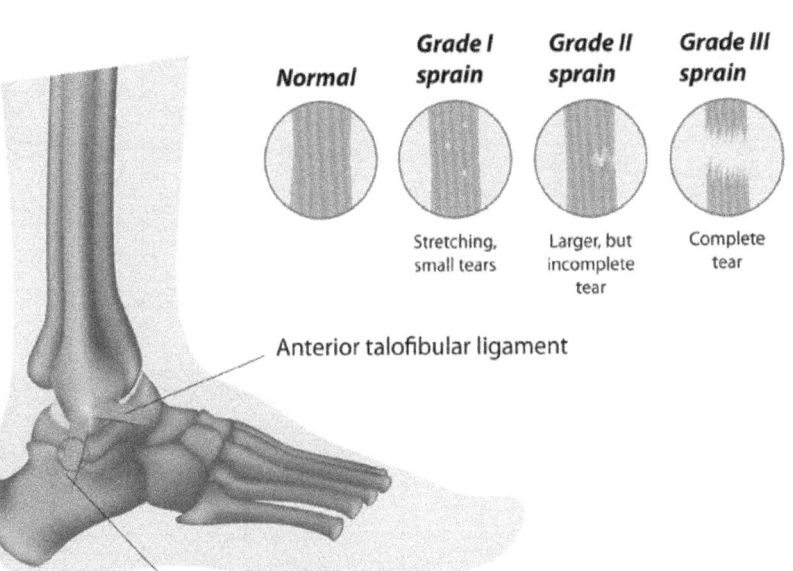

Grade I, III, or II are the three types of sprains. A Grade I strain is the most common. It usually causes minimal damage to the ligaments and is not likely to cause instability. There will be mild swelling and tenderness at the injury site.

A Grade II strain is a partial tear in the ligament. This is typically associated with some laxity, or hypermobility. Bruising at or near to the injury site may be visible. You might feel some tenderness around the injury site. There may also be mild pain and swelling. You should keep a brace on the injured area for at least two weeks. In the best case, scar tissue will develop and compensate for the ligament's laxity. This will ensure that the joint does not become hypermobile.

For future sprains to avoid, you must have proper muscle strength and proprioception for the lower feet. Proprioception describes the body's ability to use tiny receptors located in tissues, muscles, and joints to determine its location in space. Proprioception lets you know, even if you close your eyes, what your arm's doing.

A well-trained physician, therapist or athlete can usually assess the likelihood of a sprain occurring and determine the ligaments. An Xray may be necessary to rule out other injuries such as a fibular or fifth-metatarsal fracture.

Grade III ligament tears can result from sprains. There is often significant swelling and bruising with ankle instability. A consultation with an orthopaedic specialist is recommended for any possible repair. Following surgery, it is recommended that you receive guided physical therapy.

STRAINS

As with sprains strains can also be categorized as Grade I or II.

A Grade I tear can be classified as minor strain, while a complete tear, or tear, will be classified as a grade III tear. Grade II tears are partial or complete tears. Severe Grade II or Grade III tears cause muscle weakness and can be associated with bruising at the injury site. Grade I injuries tend not to heal fully, but they are milder. You can speed up the healing process with good care and rehabilitation. While Grade II tear can often also be rehabilitated, the healing times are longer. Grade III tear may require surgical intervention.

Healing is in phases

Understanding how your body heals is essential. Also, understanding the processes that occur during different phases of healing is vital. The healing phases include bleeding, inflammation, proliferation and maturation.

To guide rehabilitation, it is important to understand the changes in the body's tissue during each phase. The phases or stages can overlap and are not mutually exclusive. You can either influence the outcome positively or negatively depending on your treatment methods.

These descriptions will help to identify the phases of healing or rehabilitation and how you can best treat them.

ACUTE-PROTECTION PHASE

The bleeding and inflammation phase of healing is closely linked to the acute phase of rehabilitation. The bleeding stage is the first sign of healing. To stop further damage, the body will respond by restricting movement via swelling and spasming (splinting).

Many important inflammatory compounds are released into the bloodstream at the site of injury during bleeding and the initial inflammation phase. This initial inflammatory response plays a crucial role in healing the area. The problem with inflammation is when it becomes severe and chronic. This can cause more tissue damage.

A soft tissue trauma is considered acute as soon as it occurs. This includes the most severe symptoms such bleeding, pain, swelling, and bleeding. It takes between two and four days for acute symptoms to appear. This time frame can change depending on how you treat the injury. Sometimes, the acute phase takes longer.

This stage focuses on protecting your injury against further damage by movement and activity. Avoid tissue mobilisation and excessive activity.

One common mistake is to use medications that could negatively impact healing. This does not allow the body to go through this entire process. I advise that you do not start anti-inflammatory medication if your swelling is too severe. While you should reduce swelling, it is important to not eliminate it entirely. Your body will go through every phase of healing and need to manage it.

SUB-ACUTE -- REPAIRPHASE

The proliferation phase often corresponds with the subacute phase. The body is progressing in healing the injury. A soft tissue injury is called sub-acute when the initial phase of acute transitions to the repair and maintenance of the injured tissues. This phase of tissue repair and rehabilitation begins approximately three to six weeks after the injury. Your body will begin to heal or create new tissues. This phase lasts for as long as six weeks.

Your body will begin to eliminate any leftover injuries. This is also the beginning of healing by bringing in nutrients and a combination of extracellular matrix and collagen to make new tissue. Angiogenesis, which is the creation of new blood vessels in order to replace the ones that are damaged, is a process known as angiogenesis.

This is the most important step in a rehabilitation plan to ensure a fast recovery. It is important to reduce the need to shield your injury from the new scar tissue that begins to grow and strengthen. It is a crucial time to give your body the resources it needs for a quick and complete healing process. Your body should be able to produce as strong scar tissue as possible, while also limiting the loss of function.

LATE STAGE – REMODELING PHASE

The remodeling or late stage often occurs in conjunction with the completion of the subacute phase of rehabilitation. During remodeling, the body continues to heal and reconstruct the damaged tissue. Healing is a process. This phase lasts between six and eight week after an injury.

This stage is when your healing tissue has reached a mature state. However, as your body stresses and strengthens around the new scar tissue, you may find it unable to handle your growing physical demands. It is essential to follow a carefully coached and rated rehabilitation plan. While it may seem as though the injury has healed, maturation phase can begin. It is crucial that you continue the treatment plan.

If the treatment plan and the injury site aren't followed up on, it is possible for the site to fail. Injury sites may become even weaker as they age, even after maturation. From the initial injury, rehabilitation must include a full recovery to strength, mobility, and equilibrium.

Your body can determine if the repaired structure is still too weak. The body will either learn to compensate or put too much stress elsewhere which can increase the chance of injury. The best rehabilitation and training will allow you to perform your daily activities safely and without risk of injury.

CHRONIC PHASE - INTENSE REPAIRS and REMODELING

The chronic phase lasts for three months. This phase may be combined with the remodeling phase up to six to twelve month after an injury. This phase corresponds with the return to sports and activities phase of the rehabilitation.

The micro-trauma you experience from daily activities or workouts is constantly affecting soft tissues. This stimulates the body's ability to repair and modify the tissue according to your needs. This is the reason people train. This is the Overload Principle. The body must maintain sufficient stimulation to "overload" the tissues and stimulate them to grow stronger. In the event of injury, the stimulus was too strong. Training should not "overload" tissues with too much stimulus. This will produce the desired training effect.

Acute Phases of Rehabilitation

A popping sound can often be heard or felt at the injury site. This is followed quickly by swelling in your ankle. This usually occurs along the lateral side of your ankle, near the bump known the lateral maleolus. The swelling may extend to the entire leg, or up to the ankle. You may also experience significant pain.

Treatment will differ depending on the severity and location of the pain. If you are unsure about the severity of the injury or suspect that it is severe (such a fracture), or are in severe pain, seek the advice of a physician, physical therapist, athletic trainer, or other qualified medical professional.

An Xray may be necessary depending on the type of injury and severity of pain to determine if there were any possible bone fractures. If there was a fracture, the first phase of treatment would likely be different. This would mean that the acute phase will take longer and you may need to immobilize for some time. It is possible that the recovery process afterward will vary slightly. However, it should generally follow this course of treatment.

The Ottawa Ankle and Foot Rules outline when and whether an injury to an ankle or foot should be evaluated with an Xray. An Xray should be taken if the patient has pain in their Malleolar Zone (see the white arrows), and any of these findings: bone tenderness or inability to bear body weight (four steps) within 24 hours after the injury. A foot Xray will be taken if there is pain in the Midfoot

Area (see black arrows). Also, bone tenderness and inability to bear any weight (four steps) are possible.

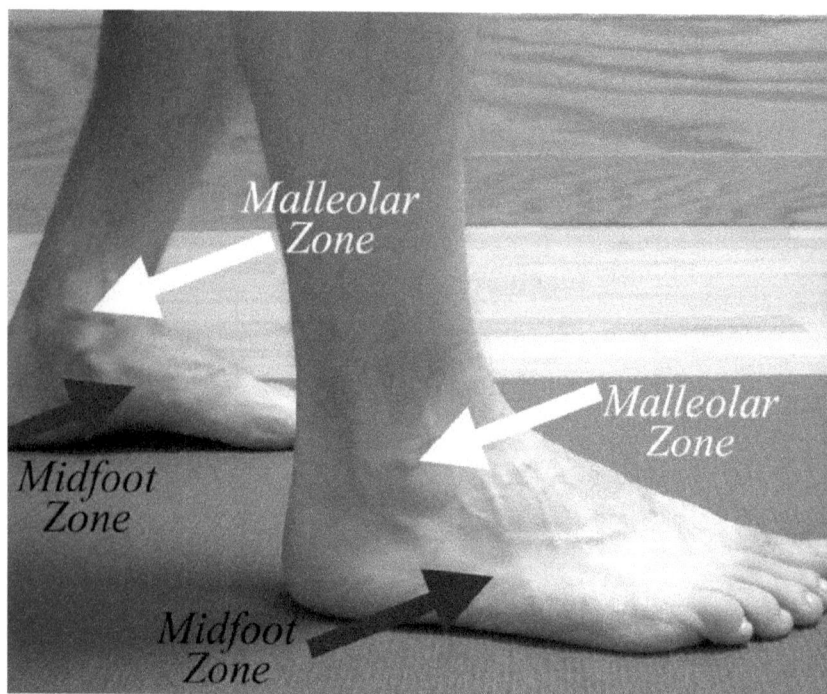

The primary goal of treatment in the acute phase, is to prevent your injury from further damage through movement, activity or other treatment modalities. An air splint, ACE Wrap, or other slip-on or laced brace may be worn to provide stability, inflammation, pain control, and pain relief for the ankle. If the injury is severe, a cast or walking boot may be necessary. A crutch or walking boot may be required to relieve the pressure placed on your ankle.

For most cases, the brace will be removed as soon as the pain subsides. The goal is to be back in full motion as soon after the injury has subsided.

For several weeks, a splint can be worn if you have a Grade 2 sprain. Your ankle and the injured ligament will likely stiffen. This will keep the ligament from becoming too stretched or loose, which can reduce the likelihood of re-injury.

You should limit your weight bearing during the initial phase. The sub-acute phase may require you to restrict your weight bearing. You can also use tape and a strap to reduce the stress on the damaged tissues.

INITIAL TRAITMENT

Following a sprain, you will need to treat it with PRICE, which stands as Protection, Rest, Ice, Compression, and Elevation.

* PROTECT: You might initially want to "protect" the injured area. This can include the use of crutches, a walking boot or cast, and/or a splint. Even a simple ACE wrap can help protect the injury site. Do not engage in any activity that could cause the injury. Don't over-rotate or move the injures.

* REST: In this case, you would not use your ankle. A crutch or crutches would be a good choice to use for walking. For your body to heal, it must rest. You must get enough rest to heal.

* ICE: Ice is applied to the ankle. For icing, you should not apply it for more than 20 minutes each hour. If you're using gel packs, don't place the ice directly onto the skin. You should exercise caution when icing people with poor circulation. A bag of frozen beans can be a great option. You can use a cold

treatment machine that circulates cool, water over the site of injury if you already have one.

* COMPRESSION: Compression can reduce and prevent swelling. If the swelling is too severe, it can lead increase in pain and slow down healing. You should limit swelling as much possible. You can use a simple ACE wrap or purchase mild over-the-counter compression socks. You can ask a friend with medical training to help you reduce swelling and bruising. Kinesiology Tape may be applied by athletic trainers or physical therapists. Or you can search online for application methods. Ankle Self-Taping Strategies is where I show you how to reduce swelling. There are many other ways to ease pain or stabilize your ankles. I have had success with KT TAPE (RockTape), Kinesiology Tape and Mummy Tape brands.

* ELEVATION means to raise the ankle above that of the heart. This allows gravity the ability to reduce inflammation and swelling. I

would normally combine the ice and compression with elevation.

The Protection Phase has three main goals. They are to reduce pain, reduce swelling, and avoid further injury. The Protection Phase increases your chances of a full healing.

* Heat causes swelling and bleeding. Avoid heat packs and saunas.

* ALCOHOL increases blood loss and swelling by thinning the blood. Too much alcohol can hinder the healing process.

* RUNING, exercising or any activity that causes injury to worsen can cause pain, swelling and bleeding. Before returning to any activity or sport, always consult a medical professional.

* MASSAGE or tissue mobilization may increase swelling and bleeding. Injured tissues can be worsened by direct mobilization. If you are not trained in proper mobilization, avoid mobilization for 48 to 72 hours. It may be beneficial to have a lymphatic or indirect

massage performed away from the injury site during the initial injury. To get the best advice about your injury, consult your physician.

*Smoking has been shown not to increase the healing response. Your healing time will be shorter if you quit smoking during recovery.

You will move out of the Protection Phase 48-72 hours after your injury. With the exception for severe injuries, the following Acute phase should not exceed seven to ten working days.

The Acute Phase of healing can overlap with the Sub Acute Phase. Understanding the Phases of healing is essential as it helps guide rehabilitation.

However, your speed of progress between rehabilitation phases will vary. Variation in healing times can be attributed to many variables, such as the severity and activity of the injury, age, current activity status and nutritional factors. It also depends on how fast your body heals.

GENTLE MOVEMENT

The ability to move gently can reduce swelling. The motion aids in healing by allowing your body to absorb nutrients at the site of injury. Your ankle should be moved as much as possible during the acute phase. Move your ankle only if it causes a slight to moderate increase in pain. This could irritate an injury and cause additional swelling and inflammation. Movement is helpful and good unless it causes severe pain.

Your ankle movement (also called plantarflexion or dorsiflexion) should be emphasized. Avoid side to side motions (also called inversion and/or eversion). It is important to return your full range or motion (ROM), as quickly as possible and without more damage. Avoid extreme movements, especially on the sides, as this can cause ligament strain or overstretchment. Maintain a range of motion that is normal and avoid extreme endings.

RANGE OF MOTION

Your ankle's range-of-motion (ROM) should be increased. Begin by working on dorsiflexion, plantarflexion, and dorsiflexion movements (the forward/backward movement of your ankle). Once your pain subsides, then you can start to move side to side.

Always start with the easiest exercise, before moving to the more challenging. It is important that exercises are pain-free and there is no more discomfort than a slight increase.

Ankle Pumps is an easy exercise to start with. Pump your ankle forward to dorsiflexion, plantarflexion, and dorsiflexion. You can do 10-15 repetitions on both feet.

The strap can be used to dorsiflex and stretch the Achilles tendon. It is slightly more difficult. Use a strap to ensure that there is no more than a slight increase or decrease in pain when performing any of the suggested movements and stretches.

To do the Foot and Ankle Strap with a Strap, wrap a strap or belt around your foot. Pull your ankle, foot, and toes upwards towards your shin, until you feel a stretch at the bottom of your foot. You can do this stretch barefoot but shoes are not necessary. Each leg should be held for approximately 1-2 minutes. Repeat this process 2 to 3 times daily.

SUPPLEMENTATION

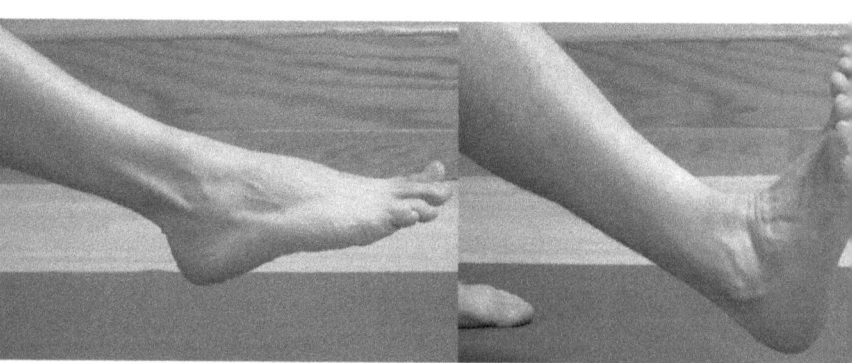

CapraFlex from Mt. Capra. CapraFlex organic glucosamine/chondroitin supplements also include a herbal/spice formulation to naturally decrease inflammation. Although it takes some time for it to build up in the body, it should not disrupt the critical inflammatory healing elements.

CapraFlex I highly recommend to anyone trying to recover from an injury, or to prevent injury during high-level performance. It's something that I have used personally.

CapraFlex could cause side effects in some blood thinners. Check with your physician if CapraFlex is prescribed to you. CapraFlex may also contain goat protein, which is a problem if you have an allergy to goat-based products. (I prefer goat protein products because they are the most similar in size to our own.

Hammer Nutrition's Tissue Rejuvenator also contains chondroitin (glucosamine) and chondroitin. There are also a variety of spices, herbs and enzymes in Tissue Rejuvenator to support tissues and minimize inflammation. I recommend CapraFlex OR Tissue Reminerator.

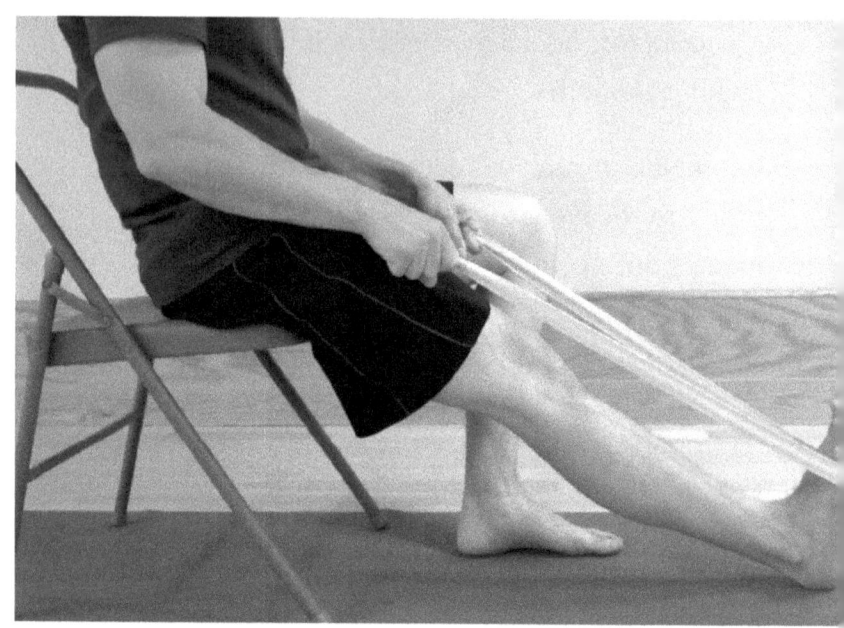

CapraColostrum by Mt. Capra is also made from goat-based ingredients. Colostrum refers to the first milk produced after a woman gives birth. It is rich with immunoglobulins as well anti-microbial and growth factors. It strengthens the intestinal lining and prevents or heals leaky gut. Colostrum may also be useful in helping people to exercise in hotter weather. Colostrum can help boost immunity, improve intestinal health, and make it easier to heal faster.

CapraColostrum can either be used alone or in combination with CapraFlex OR tissue rejuvenator. These supplements are recommended as a recuperative strategy. It is worth trying the 30-day protocol for your first 30 days. You may want to continue taking the supplements if they are assisting your recovery. This protocol is implemented as part of a prevention strategy in high intensity training.

HEALTHY EATING

Your body requires nutrients to function at a high level. Eat for performance. Your food is your fuel. The old adage "Food is your fuel" is very true. You are what is in your mouth. Avoid processed foods whenever possible. Nutrient rich foods are best. No empty calories. Avoid sugary foods, and include more healthy protein and healthy oil in your diet. In order to ensure that all hormone functions are supported and the brain and nervous systems are well-nourished, it is vital that you eat a healthy diet. For muscle health and development, it is important to get enough protein.

PAIN RELIEF

* In certain cases, an electronic device like a TENS can also be used to provide pain relief. TENS is an acronym for TRANSCUTANEOUS, ELECTRICAL, NERVE STIMULATION. A TENS unit works by the assumption that the skin and sensory nerves can transmit sensation faster than pain fibres. This means that you can reduce the perception of pain by using an electrical device like a TENS. TENS devices can be used as a short-term treatment to manage pain. Discuss your concerns with your healthcare provider.

* TOPICAL AALGESICS. There are many topical treatments that can be used for pain. Arnica Rub (an eminent herbal rub) is my favorite to relieve stiffness and pain. Biofreeze is also a great option. Use generously. They may help with the pain, but they do not get to the root cause. Consider icing to reduce pain.

* ORAL MAGNESIUM. Mag Glycinate pills are recommended. Additional magnesium can help reduce pain, especially at night. It's also great for reducing muscle soreness. I recommend that you start with 200 mg (before going to bed) and then increase the amount as needed. You should be aware that too much magnesium can cause diarrhea. Mag Glycinate oral is the most absorbable. Thorne Research Magnesium Citrate or magnesium oxide, while not as absorbable can still be of benefit.

Magnesium is well-known for its ability to decrease pain and soreness. You can try a magnesium-ice soak. Add the magnesium flake to cold or icewater. Although the magnesium flakes may not absorb as well as the water, it will still give you the benefits of the magnesium and cryotherapy (using extreme temperatures as medical therapy). Other options include Epsoak Epson Salz or Ancient Minerals magnesium bath flakes. While magnesium flakes work well, they are much more expensive than Epson sea salt.

* ACUPUNCTURE. Acupuncture is something I personally love. It's extremely useful in treating all sorts of medical conditions. It has been shown that acupuncture is very effective in pain relief. It addresses multiple layers, which can make it particularly effective for pain relief. Acupuncture treatments may help to reduce initial swelling.

* SPEAK OUT FOR HELP. A healthcare professional can provide competent advice if you are uncertain about the severity of the injury or suspect a more serious injury (such as fracture) or are experiencing severe pain. Look for a skilled and competent physician, therapist, athletic trainer, or sports chiropractor who specializes working with athletes.

The American Physical Therapy Association can help you locate a physical therapist in the area. You can get physical therapy advice from most states without needing a referral from a physician. However, it's a good idea for you to check with your physician.

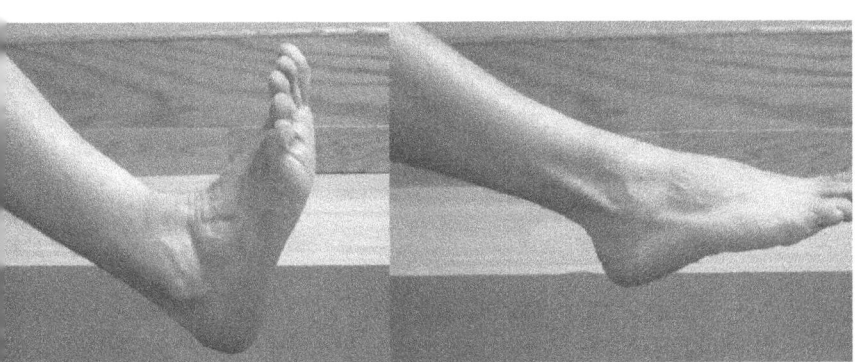

REHABILITATION RECAP FOR THE ACUTE ANKLE SPRAIN

PRICE (Protect.

Slowly, try to regain your limited mobility and range-of-motion (ROM), in your ankle. Take pain-relieving measures and rest.

Your body needs nutrients and quality food to heal. You can supplement your body with nutrients to speed up recovery.

Do your best to be active but do not stress the injury. You might need to restrict mobility or weight bearing temporarily if the injury has become more severe.

Before moving to the subacute phase, ensure the following:

* You should have equal weight on both your feet to be able stand and not feel any pain.

* Lower leg swelling is manageable.

* You are able to walk, but the ankle will likely be stiff.

* There are no other injuries that require medical management.

An ankle sprain's initial acute phase can last up to seven days. Some cases are more severe and may require longer recovery times. If you're unsure how to move forward with your rehabilitation, don't hesitate to ask for help.

Rehabilitation: Intermediate (Subacute) Phase

Your injury occurred three to ten business days ago. This phase of rehabilitation can take anywhere from 7 days to several weeks. Then, you will move on to the final phase.

The sub-acute rehabilitation phase will correspond with other phases of healing such as the repair or proliferation phase, which can last up six weeks. Near the end of the intermediate/sub-acute rehabilitation phase, you may even be in the remodeling phase or maturation phase of healing. This will begin between six and eight weeks after injury. It will continue for three to four months as your body continues healing and remodeling the injured tissue. Healing is a process. Sometimes, the phases of healing can overlap. These phases are more closely related to rehabilitation phases, but they will differ.

Are you ready?

Before initiating the rehabilitation protocol to the intermediate (subacute) phase, it is important to be able to:

Keep your weight equal on your feet so that you don't feel an increase in ankle pain.

* Take a walk, even though your ankle might be stiff.

This phase will include active treatment and activity. Each person's journey to recovery is different. Your recovery time will vary depending on how much you spend on each exercise.

During this phase you will:

* Restore your normal walking speed

* Expand your range and motion (ROM).

* Start gentle resistive exercises.

* Begin proprioceptive balance exercises. Proprioception (a fancy name for your nervous system that recognizes the position of your body in space) This is how you can tell what your extremities doing, even if you don't see them.

You can continue to use the strategies described in the Acute Phase. These include rest, supplementation, pain relief, swelling management (PRICE), and rest. Moving from the intermediate (sub-acute), phase of rehabilitation to the next is always dependent on your symptoms.

WALKING

The goal is to normalize your walking. This is achieved by having a proper foot strike. This includes rolling onto the feet into full weight bearing and propelling forward with a tee off. It is important to normalize your gait pattern and not increase your pain or cause excessive swelling.

Walking is a good habit to maintain.

If you are using a crutch to weight your foot, then you can start increasing your weight while walking. You can continue using the crutch until you feel able to walk normal and without limping. Your goal is to walk normal until you no longer have a limp. It is better not to use the crutch as a weight-bearing device on the leg or foot for more than necessary to achieve a near normal walk or gait.

RANGE OF MOTION

Your ankle's range-of-motion (ROM) should be increased. Begin by working on dorsiflexion, plantarflexion, and dorsiflexion movements (the forward/backward movement of your ankle). Once your pain subsides, then you can start to move side to side. It is vital to regain full dorsiflexion. In most cases, you should put more emphasis on regaining your dorsiflexion.

Always start with the easiest exercise, before moving to the more challenging. It is important that exercises are painless with minimal discomfort.

RECOMMENDED EXERCISES

Ankle pumps are a quick and easy exercise. Pump your ankle forward to dorsiflexion, plantarflexion, and plantarflexion. You can do 10-15 repetitions on both feet.

Ankle Alphabet, another recommended exercise, is also recommended. Imagine that you're a pen and move your foot, ankle, and toes. Capital letters are used to create the alphabet. Perform this task 1-2 times daily.

Stretch your calf gently (as shown in the video). You should feel a slight discomfort or increase in pain during these stretches. Start with the strap. As your pain permits, you can move to standing.

Foot and Ankle Stretches with a Strap

* Attach a strap (or belt), around the foot. Pull your ankle, toes, and foot up toward your shin until there is a stretch in the bottom or your calf muscles. You can do this stretch barefoot but shoes are not necessary.

* Repeat the above for at least 1-2 minutes on each leg 2 or 3 days per day.

Calf Stretch - Gastrocnemius

Stand tall and lean against the wall or counter. Then, bend your front knee so that the lower leg is slightly stretched. Maintain an upright posture.

* Your back should be straight with your heel on top.

* Perform 3 reps on each side for 30 seconds.

Calf Stretch - Soleus

* Stand tall and lean against the wall or counter. Then, bend your front knee so that you feel a gentle stretch in the lower leg. Maintain an upright posture.

* Bend your back and place your heel on to the ground.

* Perform 3 reps on each side for 30 seconds.

Self-Subtalar Mobilization

Attach a thicker, more flexible mobility or exercise band onto a stable surface. Place the band below the affected ankle with the affected leg behind you. You will feel a gentle stretch at the back of your lower legs if you bend your front knee. Remain upright.

* Bend your back knee while keeping your heel on a flat surface. Gently rotate while you feel a stretch along your calf.

* Hold the position for 30 seconds and then do 3 more repetitions.

MOBILITY/COMPRESSION BADS FOR ANKLE SPRAIN

Mobility bands, like Rogue Fitness VooDoo X Bands as well as EDGE Mobility Bands for self-treatment, are gaining popularity. The mobility bands improve blood flow and speed up healing. Mobility bands can also reset certain receptor cells within the muscle tissue that cause excessive muscle tightness. There are many methods and theories on how to use the mobile band. The exact technique used will vary depending on the injury.

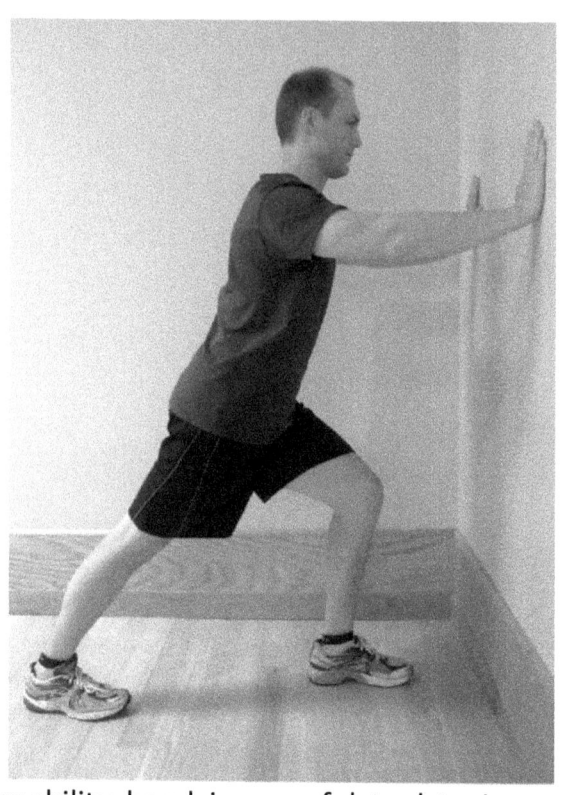

A mobility band is a useful tool to increase range of motion (ROM), decrease swelling, and reduce pain after an ankle injury. In order to not restrict blood flow, the key is to wrap your mobility band with less pressure than you would in other treatment methods. The stretch should be less than 25% on the mobility band.

The entire treatment should be completed in a matter of minutes. The treatment should be stopped if you experience any sensations such as tingling or excessive pain, or numbness. The mobility band should be removed. You should move your ankle while doing ankle dorsiflexion, plantarflexion.

This can be used for high ankle sprains. The circumferential tape technique can be used if the tape has not been damaged. Please refer to Ankle Self Taping Strategies - High Ankle Sprains - Circumferential Tabing.

I wouldn't recommend using mobility bands for any type or aggressive deep compression if you have any form of blood-clotting disorder.

Ankle Sprains/Strains - Mid Foot Variation – Part 1

Wrap the mobility belt with 25% stretch, starting from the middle of your foot. The mobility band's end should be tucked inside the wrap.

* Stand with your ankle straight and allow your legs to freely move.

Mid Foot Variation – Part 2

* Keep the mobility band in place. Pump your ankle forward and back for maximum motion in all directions.

* Perform for about 30-60 seconds.

ANKLESELF-TAPING Strategies - POSTERIOR BUIBULAR GLIDE

Part 1 - Posterior Fibular Slide

* Place the athletic tap slightly in front the injured ankle's medial malleolus. The malleolus (large bump on the ankle) is actually part or the fibular bones.

* Hold the tape about a half inch in front of your bone. Gently pull it backwards with all the force you can.

Part 2 - Posterior Fibiular Glide

* Tend not to pull the tape backwards. Wrap the tape around your leg. Pull the malleolus towards the back to maintain tension.

You can use extra tape if you feel the tape is slipping or moving. If the tape is useful, you should experience an immediate decrease in pain. You should be cautious when tape is applied to swollen feet.

ANKLE SELF - KINESIOLOGICAL TAKING EDEMA - SWELLING

Kinesiological Taping – Step 1

* Turn the Kinesiological tap over and cut the strips to approximately quarter inch width along the lines. The last inch should not be cut.

Kinesiological tape - Step 2

* Trim the uncut corners so it doesn't catch on your clothes.

Kinesiological tape - Step 3

Apply the anchor (the base of one inch) to the area that is most affected by swelling. Use only slight tension. The strips should be laid gently, without tension, over the affected area.

* Kinesiological tapes are adjustable depending on severity and how effective they work for you.

Kinesiological tape - Step 4

* Depending upon the area being swollen you may need to place several layers of tape.

* This technique may be combined with other forms Kinesiological Taping, such as the Circumferential tape for high ankle sprains.

ANKLE SELF - CIRCUMFERENTIAL TAKING - HIGH ANKLE SPRAINS

Circumferential taping - Step 1.

* Sit down so that no weight is passing through your foot or ankle. Make sure your ankle is in a neutral, 90-degree position.

Apply the tape to the ankle. You will only need to wrap the tape once or twice around each ankle. Be sure to wrap just below the ankle malleoli.

Step 2 - Circumferential taping

* If wrapping the tape around, you should not feel any tension if you're sitting down. When you stand up, tension will develop. Make sure the tape is secure but not too tight. It shouldn't cause any pain or affect blood flow.

*The tape must be worn for at most six weeks to ensure optimal rehabilitation. Without the tape, you can't eat any food.

TAPING TO SKIN CARE

WEARING

* Prior to applying, trim the edges.

By rounding the corners, you can ensure the edges do no catch on clothing and don't come up too soon.

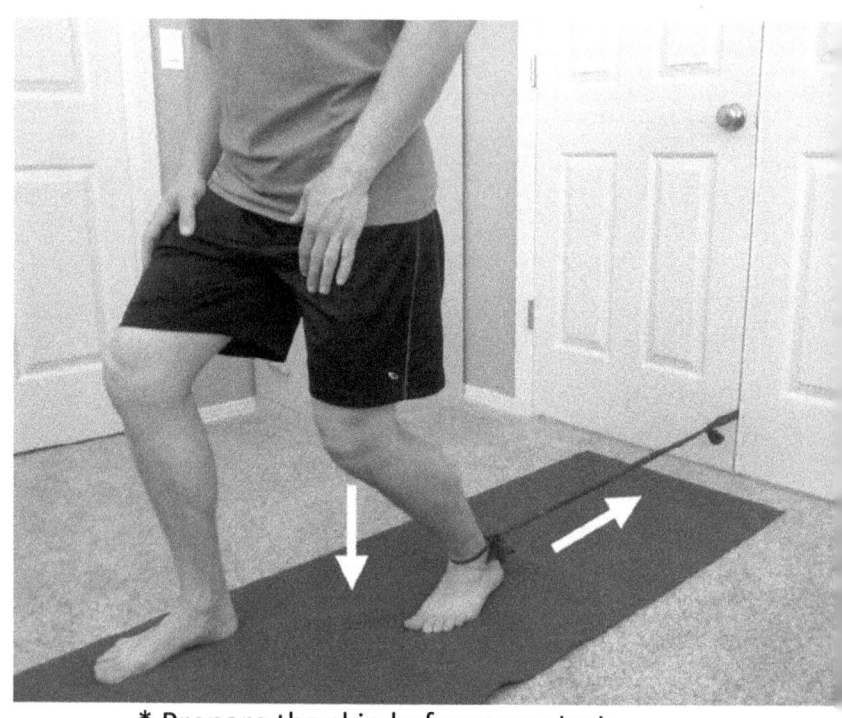

* Prepare the skin before you start.

Make sure that the skin is clean, dry and free of body oils and lotions. A skin preparation fluid that protects the skin may be recommended. Allow it to dry before applying the tape. It is possible to remove body hair using scissors or clippers. However I do not recommend shaving before applying the tape, as it can be irritating to the skin.

* The tape is flexible and can be worn for several consecutive days.

The tape can be kept on for approximately 4-5 days. Most people can wear the tape for at least a week. Your skin and the area taped may influence this. Talk with your physical therapy professional about this.

* Put the tape on your head and shower.

The tape is waterproof and resistant to water. The tape can be worn while you shower or swim. The tape can be dried once you're out of the water.

REMOVAL

* Move the tape in the direction that hair grows.

If you pull your hair out, the tape will give off a "waxing" effect.

* Remove the tape from your skin.

Do not pull the tape off like a Band Aid. As you remove the tape, peel it back and gently work the skin. Removing the tape from the body at an angle of 90 degrees can expose layers of skin. This can lead to redness and irritation.

* Moisturize your skin.

Apply a light moisturizer to your skin just like you would in your day-to-day care.

ANKLE RESISTANCE WORKOUTS - USE THE ELASTIC XERCISE BANNER

Sub-acute rehabilitation for ankle sprains/strains involves strengthening the muscles controlling the ankle and foot. Theraband Exercise Band is used in the following basic ankle strengthening activities. The red band can be seen and is one the most gentle resistances. Keep at it until you can use the green band or higher for additional resistance. While the movements may seem a bit jittery at times, you should concentrate on slow controlled movements. Your goal is to improve strength and motor control.

* An adult friend or relative may be able to hold the elasticband (but not tie it to a desk as shown). It is important to remember that elastic bands must not be tied to moving objects.

* Remember to take slow, controlled movements during these exercises. While performing these exercises, you should feel a mild or moderate increase in pain.

* Start only with the up/down motions (plantarflexion/dorsiflexion). As your pain decreases, and your range increases, you can then move to inversions and eversions with the exercise bands. Stop if your pain is severe.

Elastic band plantarflexion

* Position your foot in neutral.

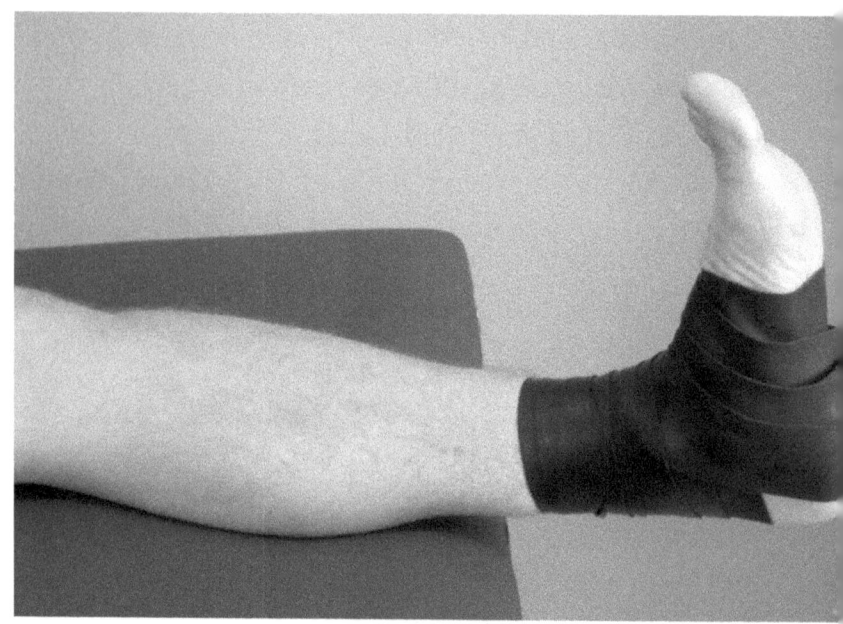

* The elastic bands can be used to raise your foot toward you, similar to a standing leg stretch.

* Sit straightened and attach an elastic band to your feet. Then press your foot down and forward. You can slowly return to your starting position, but you must be careful and keep your hand on the controls.

* Perform 2 sets, 10-15 repetitions, 1-2x per day on both feet.

* Your foot could be held on a chair or stool with your heel on the ground.

Elastic Band Dorsiflexion

* Stand with your foot slightly bent.

* Sit on a chair and hold an elastic band at your feet. Draw your foot upward.

* Perform 2 sets, 10-15 repetitions, 2-3 times per day on each foot.

* Your heel might rest on the ground or be suspended on a stool or chair.

Inversion of Elastic Band

* Position your foot in neutral.

* Sit on a chair and place an elastic band around your foot. Pull your foot inward.

* Perform 2 sets, 10-15 repetitions, 2-3 times per day on both your feet.

* Your heel might rest on the ground or be suspended on a stool.

Elastic Band Eversion

* Position your foot in a neutral place.

* Sit straight and use an elastic band to attach your foot. The elastic band will draw your foot toward the side.

* Perform two sets of 10-15 repetitions on both feet.

* Your heel may be resting on the ground or suspended on a stool or chair.

As your pain improves, standing heel and/or toe elevates can be done. But you must not feel more than a mild rise in pain. At first, you may not use the step. Then, gradually, you will start to use the step (as seen below). Be slow and controlled. Tape can be used to perform all exercises.

Heel Raises - Starting Position

* The heel lift is an essential exercise. Concentrate on eccentric control. That is, when the muscle contracting or lengthening eccentrically.

* For this exercise, the starting point is to place your feet on the tips of your toes. The most important part is to slowly lower your heels. Slowly lower the heels for several seconds. If your pain continues to worsen, you can stop this exercise.

* I recommend taking 1 second up when you are coming down and 5 seconds when you are going up.

Heel Raises - Ending Position

* Normal strength should allow you to do 25 repetitions on one leg while holding a balance bar for minor balance. Start slowly so that you don't aggravate any painful areas while working on your ankles and plantarflexion strength.

* Perform both feet at first. Do 10 repetitions at one time. You can do 3 sets of 10 repetitions daily. Start to move on to the next foot and increase the repetitions.

FOOT EXERCISES

It is vital to work on the intric muscles of your foot and ankle. This is one example of how to do this. You could also try to pick up marbles from your toes.

Foot Intrinsic muscle Strengthening

* Lay a towel flat on the ground. Best results are achieved with a non-carpeted, slick floor. Grab and roll the towel using your toes. Grab the towel with your toes, and extend them.

* Perform three sets each of 10 repetitions on each leg once per day

ANKLE RESISTANCE WORKOUTS - OTHER STRENGTHENING

It is crucial to increase the weight bearing at the ankle while you do strengthening exercises. Squatting is a good way to not only increase your leg strength but also to promote greater ankle mobility. It is possible to start with a partial squat and not be capable of moving into a full one. Instead, do a partial-squat using a chair (as shown to the right). Start with two sets of 10-15 repetitions.

Your range of motion (ROM), pain and discomfort will reduce, so you can work on your squat further (as shown to the right). Start with 2 sets of 10-15 repetitions. The goal of ROM is to maintain a normal movement pattern. (Finish the Rehabilitation Phase by not adding any weight or resistance to the movement until you reach the Return-to-Full Activity and Sport phase.

Take note of the difference in the ankle's range of motion during partial squats and full squats. For proper positioning of your knee and ankle, make sure your knee is aligned with the second toe.

It may also be beneficial to use the posterior fibular slide taping technique to improve your ankle's motion and your ability walk normally and to squat. (Please refer Ankle Self-Taping Strategy - Posterior Fibular Glaze. Use the tape before performing weight bearing activities such as walking, lifting your toes and squatting.

If you are recovering after a high ankle injury and are using the circumferential taping to help you, please ensure that it's in good condition for all weight bearing activities. (Please see Ankle Self Tapping Strategies - Circumferential taping for high ankle sprains.

INITIAL BLANCING AND PROPRIOCEPTION EXERCISES

Proprioception and balance exercises are important components of the rehabilitation program. Balance can not only assist you in rehabilitation and recovery but it can also reduce your risk of reinjury.

As the pain subsides, your balance will improve and you will be able to stand on one side of the foot more easily. As you make progress, balance will become more important (this is covered in more detail in the final stage.

Standing on One Foot and Finger Tips

* For added support, you might need to hold your hand or a finger on a countertop at first.

* You shouldn't allow your body to wobble or wiggle excessively.

* Balance by using your fingertips. This exercise shouldn't cause any discomfort or pain beyond a mild increase.

Standing on one Foot

* Normal is the ability of holding the object for up to 30 seconds, with the eyes closed at the beginning and the eyes closed at the end.

* Perform for 30 seconds, 2-3 repetitions per day.

OTHER TREATMENT OPTIONS

There are many options to choose from for alternative treatment methods or modalities during the sub-acute stage. Each treatment method is appropriate for your rehabilitation. Every person is different. You may want to seek out additional rehabilitation assistance during this phase.

This eBook is intended to provide guidance on how to safely return to work after a ankle sprain. It is possible to successfully work through a rehabilitation plan for most ankle sprain cases. Sometimes, however, additional assistance may be needed or requested. Different rehabilitation professionals may have different approaches to rehabilitation. There are many treatment options.

Other options for treatment include:

* LOCAL MODALITIES. Local modalities may be used to help reduce pain or stimulate the natural healing response through energy modulation and nutrient delivery. These include ultrasound, electrical stimulation, infrared light, magnets or magnetic field use and temperature modulation (such like contrast baths). These modalities provide short-term benefit that can be used to introduce longer-lasting techniques such as exercise prescriptions that include strength, balance, range of motion, and other benefits.

This passive treatment will provide immediate relief for many clients. But, it's important to remember that these modalities can be compared to NSAID or analgesic medication. It provides temporary pain relief or inflammation relief, which allows you continue to live comfortably until you feel better.

* MANUAL TRADITIONS. For the initial relief of pain and swelling, hands-on manual techniques may be useful. Some techniques may also promote better nutrient transfer and exchange to increase the healing response. Manual techniques include soft tissue mobilization, massage; IASTM(instrument assisted soft tissues mobilization); joint mobilization methods; acupuncture; dry needling techniques.

Joint stiffness and laxity may be an outcome of injuries to the ligament, muscle, tendon or adjacent muscles in the case ankle sprains/strains. A physical therapist with a lot of experience in regaining joint motion can be helpful, but this is not required in all cases. The ultimate goal of a physical or rehabilitation professional is to guide you through rehabilitation.

The American Physical Therapy Association can help you locate a physical therapist in the area. The majority of states allow physical therapy advice to be sought without the referral of a physician. But it's a good idea for you to get your physician's approval.

* EXERCISE PRICING. Research has shown that exercising prescription is the best method to speed up recovery, reduce pain and improve your post injury function. Some exercises include strengthening exercises and specific stretching. Others may be targeted at injury sites and localized. Barbell training, proprioceptive or balance retraining, biomechanics correction and sport-specific rehab are all possible.

REHABILITATION RECAP FOR THE SUB-ACUTE ANKLE SPRAIN

Keep on using PRICE (Protect.

When you get to full range of motion (ROM), rest and use pain relievers as needed. Dorsiflexion ROM should be your first priority. You must remember that your body needs nutritious food to support its healing process. Supplementation is a way to make sure your body gets the nutrients it needs to heal quickly.

The intermediate phase is when you should be able walk without assistance. After long days or heavy usage, swelling is likely. You should feel no pain. During this period, compression stockings may be worn. You may continue with your taping methods in general. Use the circumferential taping method for at most six to eight more weeks.

Now it's time to go to the final stage of your rehabilitation after you have regained near-normal walking. Your pain levels should not be too high. You should feel able to do the basic exercises (as described in the Intermediate (Sub Acute) Phase of

Rehabilitation), without any pain or difficulty. The final stage is a complete return to daily life and, eventually, all athletic or sport activities.

While you should be active in the sub-acute period, don't be too stressed about the injury. It should be possible to resume your normal daily activities. You might need to use the brace occasionally during active periods or when you're on your feet all day.

Before you are able to move into the sub-acute stage of rehabilitation and return to full activity or sport, ensure that these things are in place:

* You should feel able to balance on one side of the injured leg.

* Only intermittent swelling occurs around the ankle, lower leg and foot. It occurs most often at night, after long periods of activity, or towards the end.

* You can light jog without feeling pain or instability in your ankles.

* There are no other injuries that require medical management.

The sub-acute phase, depending on the severity and extent of injuries to the tissues, can last anywhere from one week up to six months. Do not hesitate to seek professional guidance if in doubt about the best way to proceed with your rehab.

Sport and activity at its fullest

The most exciting part of physical therapy is helping people return to their normal activities and functions. There are many different activities and exercises that can be performed to restore functional use of the ankle.

Every individual will move through a rehabilitation plan in a different manner. Each person will progress through a rehabilitation plan in a different way. To make it clear, I offer a generic treatment plan, which can be modified to meet your specific needs.

In the final stage, you can return to your daily activities. This is when you try to minimize the possibility of the sprain happening again.

At this stage of your recovery, you should:

* Be able to walk normally and pain-free

* Lightly jog with no pain or feeling of instability

Running and other side-to–side activities can cause pain. While not contra-indicated for these activities, they should be limited unless you are wearing a slip-on brace or using taping techniques to aid in stability.

This initial stage of rehabilitation focuses primarily on strengthening and stabilizing the ankles and feet, and addressing balance deficiencies. This begins with static exercises and activities. The process eventually progresses to dynamic strength, balance, mobility activities. The rate at which one moves through this phase is variable. You need to go at your own pace.

If your ankle begins to hurt or feel unstable, you should reduce your activity levels and keep going with the strategies in the Intermediate (Sub-Acute Phase) of Rehabilitation. Continue to work on the activities that don't cause pain and discomfort once the pain subsides.

The following treatment plan includes exercises to improve strength and balance, as well mobility drills and full-athletic simulation drills. Each category is listed in the easiest to most difficult order. If you don't master the first one, you shouldn't move onto the next.

STRENGTH

* Continue with the Ankle Resistance Exercises. The red bands are one of the most gentle resistances. Keep at it until you have the ability to use the red band or more.

* Heel/Toe Raises - A normal amount of strength should allow you to do 25 heel lifts in a row, with very little assistance from a countertop. If you are able to perform 25 heel

raises only with one foot, then your calf strength should be normal.

Heel Raises

* At first, keep your feet flat on ground. This will become easier as you get more comfortable with using a step.

* You can do 10 repetitions at one time.

Heel Raises - Starting Position

* The heel lift is a crucial exercise. Concentrate on eccentric control. That is, when the muscle contracting or lengthening eccentrically.

* For this exercise, the starting point is to place your feet on the tips of your toes. Slowly lowering your heels is crucial. Slowly lower your heels for several seconds. If your pain continues to worsen, you can stop this exercise.

* I recommend taking 1 second to rise and 5 seconds to descend.

Heel Raises - Ending Position

* Start slowly to ease the pain.

* Perform both feet at first. Do 10 repetitions at one time. You can do 3 sets of 10 repetitions daily. Start to move on to the next foot and increase the repetitions.

Heel Raises - One Leg

* Perform 25 repetitions on one leg while holding a balance bar for minor balance. Start slowly to avoid aggravating the pain area while you strengthen your ankles and plantarflexion.

* You can do 10 repetitions at one time.

One Leg Partial Sweat

This particular exercise will improve strength in the calf and ankle, quadriceps and hip.

* At first you may have to place your finger tips on a countertop or a wall.

* Don't use your hands for balance. The one-leg squat on your tips toes is a tough

variation, and involves more activation of the calves.

* Begin by doing 2 sets of 10 repetitions. Next, you can move on to 3 sets with 10 repetitions.

Clock/Star Exercise

* This exercise improves strength, balance and proprioception when done correctly. To reach your non-affected side's tip toe, stand on your injured foot. Your starting point or center of your foot will be reached according to the hands on the clock. It could take you from 1 o'clock up to 6 o'clock (clock-wise), or 12 hours to 6 o'clock (counter-clock-wise), depending on the foot. Slowly perform the routine from three to five time.

Single Leg Balance with Mini Squat - The Star Drill

* In order to understand how the knee works, it is important that we also address stability and balance. This exercise will be performed on two legs. Next, you will stand on the

injured leg. You will slowly move the leg that is not injured as detailed below. Maintain your balance while reaching for the non-injured leg. As you reach further, your injured knee will be bent. Your goal is to keep balance, reach further, and keep the patella (knee cap), straight ahead.

* The exercises will be performed in sequence. To touch your toe, then go back to standing on one leg. Next, repeat the process. After completing all three positions, you will continue to work your way up until you reach the end.

Old age begins at 27

According to physiology we are taught that age 27 is the end of life. This is due to two main factors.

First, enzyme production decreases drastically after age 27. Dr. William Wong, an expert in systemic enzyme therapy has extensively discussed the impact of this drop-off and how it can affect health. Enzymes are extremely important. They act as catalysts in chemical reactions. Without enzymes things would move in the body like molasses. You would not be able function well. In fact, it would be impossible to function.

The human body has over 3,000 enzymes. These enzymes play a role in more than 7,000 chemical processes, so they are important. Enzymes are commonly thought to be involved in digestion. However, their primary function is the growth and repair tissue. They are found in such high quantities when we are young. This is also why injury heals so quickly.

Our knowledge also shows that your anabolic hormonal levels are at their lowest point in your twenties and continue to drop. One of the hormones that falls is testosterone. Testosterone plays an important role in muscle strength. The higher your chances of getting injured, the more fragile you are.

Growth hormone is another hormone which will increase lean mass and play a major role in collagen production. As collagen, you can think of it as the scaffolding which makes up your connective tissues like bones, tendons ligaments and skin. A fifth of your body is composed of protein and a third of it is collagen.

It is obvious that your quality of connective tissue will decrease as your growth hormone levels decline. An example of this is the aging of skin. The production of collagen decreases with lower levels of growth hormones.

The benefits of optimal hormone levels are undeniable. They can help you avoid injuries both in and out the gym. Stay seated, hormone testing will be discussed later.

Don't Let Your Bathtub Overflow

One hormone that does not seem to diminish with age is cortisol. There are many stressors that we face every day. Every day, we are subject to numerous stressors: chemical, physical, emotional, psychological, as well as environmental.

All stressors can be daily events, such as getting hit by a driver, having a disagreement with a spouse or coworker, losing to your favorite sports team, and so forth. Research has shown that psychological stresses, whether they are life-event or perceived stress, can hinder healing and recovery from resistance training.

A low-level infection or food intolerance can also occur. If you eat the same foods over and over, especially protein-rich foods, your body may perceive it as a stressful event and release cortisol.

A temporary increase in cortisol level isn't a problem. But, it can make a difference if you have chronically high levels. High levels of cortisol are catabolic. It breaks down muscle tissue in order to get energy. The more muscle you have the less you can do to prevent injury.

Your body can be described as a bathtub. Stressors can be viewed as taps in your bathtub. You will need to reduce the amount of training you do if your financial taps are blazing. In other words, you must reduce the amount you train during high stress situations like when you move, divorce, exam, sickness, or even death. Otherwise, your body may make it difficult to reduce training.

Hydration Extremes are to be avoided

A common stressor for many athletes is dehydration. Even a mild level of dehydration, only 1-2%, can make it difficult to perform at your best and increase the chance of injury.

Here's an interesting theory about aging. Think about the hydration status and how it changes from womb through tomb, or cradle into coffin. While our bodies contain 75-85% water upon entering this world, the percentage drops to between 50-60% after we leave the planet. Water loss occurs when we are in our twenties. This is due to the loss of lean mass. For example, muscle tissue has between 70-79% water. Therefore, if you are losing water as you age you may be losing muscle. In order to counter aging, it is essential that you maintain as much muscle mass and strength as possible. We'll discuss muscle atrophy more in a second, but for now, let's talk about hydration.

To ensure proper hydration, it is important to evaluate both your water intake and the quality. Quantity is important. You need to drink at most half your body weight per day in ounces. So if 200 lbs you should drink 100 ounces (or roughly 12 glasses) of water daily. To make it easy, fill three 1-liter bottles each morning and drink your quota by the end the day. The goal is 1 liter for the morning, 1 in afternoon, and 1 in evening.

Quality of water intake is another important aspect. Water that is not of the right quality will be absorbed poorly. It is vital to know the water's mineral content.

Choose filtered water over any other water as you might find trace amounts in your local water source. However, filtering out some "good" stuff will mean that you may need to put it back in. The easiest way to do this is to add a small amount of sea salt. At least 300 mg of dissolved substances (minerals), should be achieved per liter. If you find a bottle of water that has less than 300mg/L or 300ppm (parts/million) of dissolved substances, add some sea salt.

It is also important to make the water less acidic than it used to be. You can either buy expensive filters for this purpose or simply add fresh lemon juice or lime juice to your water. Although lemons and limes appear acidic on their outside, they are actually alkalizing on the inside. These fruits will not only give you flavor, but they will also help with digestion and absorption.

You should be cautious about "superhydration". However, I'm not referring to hyponatremia which is when marathoners consume excessive water. It can cause dangerously low electrolytes (many have even died from this kind of water intoxication). Instead, I mean superhydration of tissue.

Your spinal discs, which are hydrophilic, love water. So when you sleep, the water in your discs is filled with water, and when you wake up, they're swollen. It's the reason you're slightly taller after you get out of bed in morning than you are before you go to bed at nights. A superhydrated, swollen disc can lead to an 18% decrease in strength and increase vulnerability to injury.

According to Dr. Stuart McGill (a spinal biomechanist, professor emeritus, University of Waterloo), you should wait at least 50 minutes when you wake up before loading your spine. The time will allow synovial fluid which lubricates the joints to warm up, and help you prepare for activity.

Use it, or lose it

It doesn't matter if you lose your strength or not, it just applies to flexibility and strength as you get older. As you age your muscles will lose their strength and stiffen up.

Sarcopenia is a condition that can be translated as "loss of flesh", but it can also be called "muscle mortality". In other words, disuse will cause your muscle cells to die. Let's not forget an interesting fact. A 60 year old muscle cell is the same strength as one 20-year old, on a basis of gram per gram. The difference is that there is less muscle cross-sectional surface in the 60-yearold than the 20-yearold. In general, you will lose 50-60% strength between your twenties-sixties. The figure can get even more if you add speed components like Olympic weightlifting.

In terms of the stiffening effect: As we age, the avascular links between muscles and bones, also known by tendons, begin drying out. You start to lose collagen and elastin. Brooks Kubik's Dinosaur Training explains that you are "brittle".

The Golgi tendon or GTO organ is the little sensory organ that your body uses to sense this. This sends an inhibitive message to the brain, which slows you down to prevent injury. The tendon can snap if it is subjected to excessive tension or speed. This is something your body does not want to happen. It can lead to a decrease of speed, strength, or mobility.

If weight training is done correctly, it can help to counter this effect. You may be misled into believing that weight training makes you stiffer. Olympic weightlifters can do full squats without difficulty and still sustain very few injuries to their knees or low backs.

Strength training is crucial to avoid muscle atrophy. It can also increase flexibility, and not decrease it, if done properly.

Olympic weightlifters show high levels in flexibility.

(Photo by Sam Sabourin

Spreading the Truth

There are many misconceptions about stretching, especially regarding warming up. You should begin your warm-up by engaging in aerobic activity for 5-10 minute, and then continue with stretching, typically static stretching, for 5-10 additional minutes.

Research has shown that warming up this way can be counterproductive. Not only does this zap precious energy and strength, but it can also affect performance and increase the chance of injury.

Aerobic work or doing too many repetitions for any weight training exercise will increase your lactic acid level, which can hinder recruitment of high threshold motor units. Simply put, it makes you weaker, slower and more likely to sustain injury.

Also, static stretching can temporarily weaken muscle. You should all know this by now. Why is it necessary to perform static stretching prior to any activity?

If you only plan to do static activity such as isometrics during training then you should do static stretching. However, most people perform dynamic activities so it is important that their warm up be dynamic.

There are some exceptions to this rule. However, for the most part there's very little correlation between dynamic flexibility and static flexibility. This means that you can have an athlete, such as a Martial Artist, who is capable of punching you in the head but cannot touch their feet!

Relative flexibility is better than absolute flexibility. A straight leg raise with a supine position of 80-90 degrees would be considered normal. The normal limits are 80-90 degrees for a straight leg raise.

Now let's imagine that you can only manage 60-70 degrees, or lower. Is this a sign you're more susceptible to injury or something else? But it does not necessarily mean you'll be more likely to get hurt.

It's not the flexibility on both sides that is important. This means that you should compare your abilities to others. And believe it or otherwise, the side that is more flexible runs the risk of getting injured. When stretching, aim to achieve symmetry between both the left and right sides.

Fire on the Cue

An injury-causing factor is improper muscle timing. Sprinting is one example. If the hamstrings fire too soon or late during the stride phase, injury could occur. The same principle applies to weight training movements like glute-hamer raises and lunges. Your pre-workout dynamic stretching routine could benefit from adding proprioception (awareness about joint position) as an option.

This is how it works: For support, place your left arm on a wall/exercise machine and then lift your right leg to your right. In a pendulum style, increase the height of the kick. However, make sure to touch your right hand every time. This warm-up drill works well if your hamstring pulls are constant. See my book The Warm-Up to learn more about "ham kicks".

For the upper arm, punching is often done with elastic resistance. This can cause injury by making your accelerator muscles smaller than your decelerators. It is possible to get injured if you attempt to throw a real punch. When training, it is much better to have a punching bag and not free space.

It's great if your goal is to become a boxer or mixed-martial artist. If that's not your case, and you want to get your shoulders ready for lifting, then you should try the ShoulderRok by Kabuki Strong. The loadable mace allows you to do various swings and pendulums that will open up your shoulders, while also integrating your core. It's a popular choice for lifters with shoulder impingement. Give it another try.

Restores Your Body

A new car can be driven to the ground once it is purchased, but over time it will require more maintenance before you are ready to trade it in. The body can't be traded in for another car. This means that it will need to be maintained regularly if you don't wish it to go to pieces. To keep it in good condition, you'll need it to be taken to the "bodyshop" on a regular schedule.

Restoration is extremely important. Many lifters in Russia and Eastern Europe prepare for this - they train during the days and then work on restoration at night. However, in North America it's all about training. And restoration is often overlooked.

You have many options for restoration, such as salt baths or contrast showers. Let's take a closer look at some of the methods.

Contrast showers allow you to alternate between hot and cool for approximately 3-5 minutes each. You can either go whole-body immersion, where the temperature is the lowest, or concentrate on the affected area. A removable shower head can be used to place the contrast effect right on the quads if they are very sore from working out the day before.

Take a salt bath every other week. Don't be afraid to use the salts. 2 cups Epsom salt, 1 cup sea salt. Baking soda (sodium bicarbonate), to help exfoliate skin, along with any calming essential oils you like (e.g. lavender, chamomile), and a splash if apple cider vinegar, to help restore skin's natural acidity.

You can use electronic muscle stimulation while surfing the net. You can place the electrodes directly on the muscle you have been training the previous day, let's say your quads. Then, turn the unit on at a low intensity and pulse for 15-20 minutes to get blood flowing to the area. This will facilitate healing.

If you do it correctly, aerobic exercise can increase circulation and help with recovery. A lot of aerobic exercise can make you feel sick and could lead to injury. But walking may be the best thing for you!

Walking can be a form of locomotion, and it is great for weight loss. It can be quite beneficial to take a walk after eating, lunch and/or dinner, provided the weather is favorable. It is something that I highly recommend. We'll be talking a bit more about the health benefits of walking later.

Stretching is a great way of boosting your recovery. Everybody who weight trains should do some yoga at least once a week. If possible, static stretching should be performed separately from weight training. It can either be done in a small group or alone.

You can either attend a class on a particular night or view an online video to do it at your home. Or, you can just practice some poses while you watch TV. You could do a hero (or pigeon) pose if your tibialis anterior or shin muscles are tight. You can adapt the stretches to fit your particular needs.

As a self-massage, foam rolling can be done in conjunction with stretching. Foam rolling can be used to restore muscles after a workout. However, there's a lot of debate over its effectiveness. It's best to do this while you're watching TV.

These are just a few of the things you should do daily if your goal is to improve recovery and decrease your chances of being injured.

Yoga can be a good option for weight-lifters.

Take time to heal

Your muscles can be thought of as the meat in a sausage and your fascia, as the casing. The casing heals faster after trauma than the meat. Connective tissue such ligaments, tendon, and fascia can take up to seven times longer than muscle tissue to heal. This applies not only for the macrotrauma which can be caused by injury but also for the microtrauma that may occur during training. Give your tissue time.

A lot of this healing takes place during sleep. I won't go into too much detail about the importance of good sleep hygiene but I will say one thing: fragmented sleeping can be just as helpful for recovery and may even be more beneficial than continuous sleep. It doesn't mean that you have to sleep in the night. Power naps allow you to get that sleep in small amounts during the day.

A short power nap is one the best recovery boosters. You can take it anytime you have the time, but ideally after training. It doesn't have to be a lengthy commitment. A quick nap of 10 to 20 minutes will suffice.

A Chi machine is a great tool to help you take a deep sleep. This machine has ankle support pads. You just need to lie down on the floor and place your feet on the pads. The machine will then rock your legs from side to side. It comes with a remote that can control the speed of movement. This allows you to set the machine at a faster speed to stimulate the nervous and relax the nervous system.

The Chi machine creates an electromagnetic ripple effect that runs through the body. It is similar to the fins of a swimming fish and can improve circulation and lymphatic drainage. It also has a deeper effect. Your body experiences the sensation of being rocked gently by your mother and you fall asleep. The machine will turn off after 15 minutes. Once it stops, your body will naturally wake you up. It's the perfect remedy for a mid-day slump. It's worth looking into purchasing one. It is something I would highly recommend.

Ready to Lift

Research shows that athletes are more likely to be injured if they don't have enough quality sleep. The same holds true for the gym. Dr. Matthew Walker, a sleep expert says one aspect of sleep that is most affected by the decline in activity is stabilizer muscles. You need all of your muscles to function at an optimal level if you plan on lifting heavy weights.

Many devices now exist that can be used to help you measure your sleep and training readiness. They will use metrics like temperature, heart rate variability and pulse to measure this. If you have a high readiness score, then train hard that day. If you score low, then take it easy. I wish it was as simple as that.

There have been times when my readiness score was high, but I haven't done a lot of exercise. I have seen it happen with others. These devices can be helpful, but they don't always accurately reflect reality.

As you'll see, objective measures tends to prevail over subjective measures. However, it's your performance inside the gym that really matters. Many times, your warm up sets will determine if you should lift that specific day. For more information, refer to my book The Elite Trainer. If your baseline results are not satisfactory, you should stop training that day. Instead, focus on restoration. To lift in a tired state is like going into battle without your armor. Don't do it!

Stop licking the Scab

When you do any exercise, it is important to remember the golden rule: "If it hurts don't do that!" If it alleviates your pain, then do it! The question, "Does it hurt?" is only answered with a yes or no answer. If the answer is yes then stop moving! If you scratch the scab constantly, it will never heal.

My 12-year-old boy and I were having a lot of fun and my arm started to bleed. Although the injury was not serious, it did heal. However, it took about a week before it completely disappeared. My son would not have had it if he was scratched.

The healing process for tissue on the inside and outside of the body is similar to that of tissue on the outside. An example of this is after a bout with eccentric training. Research shows that a 20-yearold can recover in just five days while a sixty-year-old takes seven days. As you age, it is obvious that recovery will take longer.

We need to know the difference between the pain of soreness or injury. As a trainer, you'll be better at recognizing the difference. However, if your body is constantly hurting, that's not good news! Pay attention and listen to your body. Training through pain can cause joint deterioration. Don't do it! You can find another movement that will help the area and continue to train. You'll make progress, and your joints are going to be happy.

Think about the Orthopedics Cost

It is important to consider the long-term effects that exercises and training protocols will have on your body before you make a decision. Michael Boyle, strength coach and author of Strength Coach Michael Boyle refers to this as "the orthopedic cost" in training. In the short-term, you could pay the price for a rupture of tear or worsening of your joints.

Supramaximal excers with weight releasers (or high-impact exercise like loaded squat jumping or kipping pulled-ups) may have been acceptable at one stage, but they can quickly make you a numbing patient in an operating room. You should also avoid exercises that are too hard or too heavy, such as wide-grip bench press or press behind the neck. These types of exercises can cause injury and may not be recommended in later years. To reiterate this message, I have many additional examples that I'll be sharing throughout the book.

Boyle states, Strength training is like adding miles to your car. You can't turn back the clock. Continuous hauls over uneven terrain will reduce the vehicle's lifespan. The same thing could happen to your body. You can adapt your training to your age so that your machine runs for many years!

Be mature, as you mature

For long-term success in training, a plan is crucial. If you approach things in a random manner, you can get unplanned results or even get hurt. So you need to have a plan. But it is important to not be rigid in following the plan. Your training must be flexible. Here's one example.

Let's say that you intend to perform 5 sets of 5 reps of the back squat with 315lbs. Your first set is easy. You get five reps. You take a break and then start your second set. This time, you will get 5 reps. You were able to make it through this set, although it was harder. After resting for a few minutes, you begin your third set. But this time, you can only do 2 reps.

This is the time when you need to be mature enough for you to stop. It is dangerous to try to force two more sets because your plan calls for five sets. It's a mistake to reduce the weight for those sets. You will be weaker the next time you do it. The exercise should be stopped after 3 sets. For the next set, you should be capable of doing more than 2 reps.

Let's take a look at an alternate scenario. The same scenario as above, but with one exercise. Let's say that in the previous workout, you were able do five sets of five reps with 310lbs. It didn't pose any problem.

In other words, it felt like there was more to the tank.

Your next workout will be your mature one. You can only add 5 pounds to the bar (that's 2 1/2 lb per side), for a total 315 lbs. (This is called the "kaizen principles", an approach to creating continuous improvement through small, continual positive changes. If you are unable to complete 5 reps in your first set, then what if only 2? What should you then do?

You need to pack your gym bag and get home. You may need to take an extra day off for recovery. Do not train, instead focus on restoration. In this situation, a nap might be better than a training session. If you insist that you train even with a smaller weight, you are likely to injure yourself and will return the next workout weaker.

This is why you should be flexible with your training. This principle also applies to sick people. Use the neck rule to determine if your symptoms are higher than the neck (e.g., headache, runny nostrils, sore throat). This means that you can maintain the intensity (load) while reducing the number of sets. For example, instead 5 sets of 5 reps with 305 pounds, you'll do 2 to 3 sets with this weight. Even 1 set will be sufficient for strength maintenance. If you feel the symptoms below your neck (e.g., chest or bronchial infections, fever, extreme ache, etc. You can then rest the day and reassess the next morning.

Plan for a Remarkable Comeback

It's okay to take a few days off from some training. It's good both for the body as well as your mind. You get to rest and recover, and you return feeling refreshed and ready for the next round of weight lifting. Your training should be planned so that your peak time is just before your departure. Once you're done, take a vacation and bask in the rewards of all your hard work. Once you're back, you can start another program.

What happens if a sudden interruption occurs, and you have to suspend training for a time? It is not necessary to create a new program or go back to the beginning.

For this use the DeLorme approach. It's proven to work well. After the first workout, you'll be back at your best weights. Here's how this works.

DeLorme was a method that required three sets of 10 repetitions. In the first set you used 50% of the 10-repeat maximum (RM), 75% in the second and 100% in the third. For example, if your goal was to do 10 reps with 200 pounds, you would bench 100, 150 and 200 pounds in the first, second, third, and fourth sets.

Depending upon the extent of the layoff you may be able accomplish the task with this strategy. From there, you can continue building up. You can try the same strategy again the next time.

Even if the previous layoff saw you doing more than 4 or 5 sets, it is still a good idea to start with 3 sets in the first session. Next, work your way up through the remaining sessions. Use the 50/75/100% RM load for all rep schemes - no matter if you are doing 10 reps 8 reps or 5 reps - it doesn't make a difference! It's a sneaky way to do just one work set and warm-up sets prior.

Deload, or Deset

If you intend to continue a program or are a powerlifter, you shouldn't lift more than 3-4 times a week without a deload. Do 85% for the week after. That is how powerlifting icons like Brian Carroll and Ed Coan prevent injuries. This approach should be yours!

You don't need to deload if you plan to do new exercises every 3-4 months. If you are going to introduce a new exercise, start with a lighter body weight and work your ways up. The deload is included. Even though it might seem like you are making a small adjustment to an exercise like your grip or stance width, your nervous system will view it as "new" and you will have adjust the load accordingly.

Start at the lowest level and work your way up.

This is the type you would prefer to train in. You might reduce the number set per week as you increase the intensity. This is how it works: You start with a smaller number of sets, a lower load, and then increase the weight and decrease the sets. After every workout, start putting a bit more weight on your bar and reducing the number of sets for each exercise. You can stop counting sets after you reach half the number you had when you started. For example, 6 sets may have been a good starting point. After reaching 3 sets, add more weight to the bar and drop one set.

Although you may see a decrease in the number and intensity of work sets over time, this won't affect the overall number of sets that you do. You will require more warmup sets to reach your goals.

This training approach works extraordinarily well. It preserves a high level performance while reducing stress on your body and minimising the risk of injury.

You Should Wear the Pieces

To force two pieces of a puzzle together is just asking for trouble. Do not attempt to do any exercises or other training methods that aren't working for you. Be patient. It's possible that they did not work for you in the past.

Let's take, for instance, sprinting. For example, hill and stair sprints put too much stress on the Achilles tendon. Flat sprints can also overstress the hips. Some middle-aged men experienced a hamstring pulling after they started sprint training. However, it was not nearly as severe as the full effort. Perhaps sprinting on a stationary bike is a better option.

These injuries are more common in seniors than in younger people. Exercising in high-impact exercises that require a lot more jumping or performing movements like clap pull-ups or clap pushups can lead to injury to your Achilles tendon/rotator cuff. Do standing calf raisings or traditional push-ups, with a controlled lowering action and an explosive lifting motion. With far less risk of injury, you will reap just as many benefits in terms fast-twitch muscle fiber recruitment and power production.

Olympic lifting, a highly technical activity, is no exception. Many people struggle to master the technique. Even though it takes years to master the proper techniques for Olympic lifting, even then, not everyone can do it perfectly. You don't need to perform squats or deadlifts. Research shows that there is no injury risk and you'll get just as much power production benefit.

The high-repetition Olympic Lifts with Kettlebells are a popular trend. That's asking too much! You can quickly injure your elbows or rotator cuffs by performing high-rep cleanings and snatches using a kettlebell. Kettlebell swings can be dangerous, even if done correctly. Famous celebrity trainer, for using the "dive bomb", a rounded-back technique to perform kettlebell swings, was chastised. This is a great way of blowing your back!

Because of the high rate of injury, the British military had long ago banned kettlebell use.

Fatigue Management

While high reps coupled with short rest intervals can promote muscle endurance, improve body composition and help to increase muscle endurance, the fatigue this type training causes can cause injuries. The best way to accomplish this task is to perform sets in a staggered order, switching between lower- or upper-body exercises. We will take a look.

Let's say that you intend to perform three sets of 15 reps using two machine-based exercises. If you start with an 15RM load (e.g. 100 pounds for the chest presse and 200 pounds for your leg press), and then you do straight sets of 15 reps with 60 seconds of rest in between, your workout would look the following:

LEG PRESS SET #1: 200 LB X 15 REPS

LEG PRESS SET #2: 200 LB X 12 REPS

LEG PRESS SET #3: 200 LB X 10 REPS

CHEST PRESS SET #1: 100 LB X 15 REPS

CHEST PRESS SET #2: 100 LB X 12 REPS

CHEST PRESS SET #3: 100 LB X 10 REPS

Total workload: 11,100 lb

This is how your workout will look if you alternate between chest and leg presses using the exact same loads.

LEG PRESS SET #1: 200 LB X 15 REPS

CHEST PRESS SET #1: 100 LB X 15 REPS

LEG PRESS SET #2: 200 LB X 14 REPS

CHEST PRESS SET #2: 100 LB X 14 REPS

LEG PRESS SET #3: 200 LB X 13 REPS

CHEST PRESS SET #3: 100 LB X 13 REPS

Total workload: 11,700 lb

If you do straight sets with short rest intervals (or start with a maximum weight), the average trainee will lose between 2 and 3 reps per setting. However, if you do staggered set training, it is usually only 1 rep per session.

Staggered sets can be used to add 600 pounds to the above example. Both methods require the same time commitment. The sequence of the exercises doesn't change. However, this makes a significant impact on the total workload and reduces the chance of injury.

Overall, the math supports staggered sets that improve performance and reduce injuries.

Hasta la Vista, Free Weights

The machines could be a great choice as you age. Arnold Schwarzenegger (77) is now in his

70s and has switched to machines over free weights. Machines can be a great way of isolating certain muscles and are usually safe when used alone. But, as you'll soon discover, there's a risk.

Although Terminator may not have ended free weights for his clients, he did not end training. Instead, he switched over to machines. You can do it the same way, but don't forget that you're not an indestructible computer cyborg. If they aren't operated correctly, they will fail!

Alternatives not so innocent

Mike Israetel has a Ph.D. and is a former professor in nutrition and sport science. He believes you should do your heavy lifting by your mid-thirties. He recommends isolation and machine movements to reduce joint stress and injury as you age. This is sound advice but be aware.

Isolation moves are most commonly performed at lower weights. But, that doesn't necessarily mean there is less risk. Let's take, for instance, the lying dumbbell flying. The long lever arm means that a light dumbbell in the bottom position can be considerably heavier than a heavy dumbbell. In this case, the risk of injury could be very high. You shouldn't lift more than 10% from your maximum bench press.

Machines are not without risk. Overuse of machines, including the Smith machine can lead to what Chek, a holistic healthcare practitioner, refers to as "pattern overload". Too much pressing or squatting onto a Smith device can lock you into a pattern which can eventually cause a lot more pain to your shoulders/knees.

You may find that machines can put your body in an unforgiving position if you get too wild. If you lift too heavy a weight, the leg presses can be very destructive to your back.

As with all resistance exercises, once your body has adapted to a particular movement pattern, it's a good idea make a change. To change muscle recruitment, for example, you can adjust the position and height of the feet during leg presses.

You could also try a different machine. Leg curls can also be done standing, kneeling or lying down. There are machines to suit each position. Due to the unique resistance profile, even the same exercise can produce a different response.

Machines are responsible for about 19% of all injuries that occur in health clubs. They don't come with free weights. Make sure to adjust the machine for your specific structure. If it does not feel right, don't use it. Also, practice good form and don't be tied to one machine forever.

Do the same with free weights.

(Photo by Sam Moghadam Khamseh

Do not Run before You Crawl

Proper progressions in training are essential. A novice in training is not advised to do lunges before performing split squats and pull-ups after pulldowns. However, it is wise to start to master key movements before moving on to more challenging endeavors.

As an example, consider the step-up. Begin with a sidestep-up. Then, move onto a forward-stepping step-up.

Bottom line: If you want to avoid injury, crawl first and then run!

The Training Rulebook

Some exercises can require adjustments over time. If you are looking to improve your hips as you age, it may be worth changing how you do certain exercises.

Although a mixed grip may help you lift more weight while you are deadlifting, you run the risk of tearing your biceps in the supinated direction. You can eliminate this risk by using a pronated (double overhand) grip.

Another example is pressing. It is possible to press with a wide-grip, even midgrip, on your shoulders. But, close-grip is okay. Close-grip is somewhat misleading. Pressing too close to your thumbs will cause them to touch. On average males should have their fingers spaced at 14 inches and females at 8 inches. If you don't like the pronated grip, then you might try a neutral grasp with a Swiss or log bar, dumbbells, or dumbbells. A floor press is a better choice for your shoulders than an ordinary bench press.

While we're on this topic, most people do presses on a flat or 45-degree bench. For a long time, using the same grip angle or grip can lead to pattern overload. A regular change in the grip or angle of the bench can not only benefit muscular growth but also prevent injury.

This rulebook doesn't say that you can't make these modifications to your training. Do not be rude!

Friendly Options

Just a moment ago, we discussed how neutral grip pressing might be a more healthy option for your shoulders for the long-term. Here are some additional examples.

A bad idea is to spinal flexion and rotate against resistance. You can see the cable woodchop fitting this description. Most people do it from the hips, and not from the back. Maintain a static core position. The half-kneeling variation is "spine friendly" for woodchops. Make sure to brace your core throughout the movement.

If you are unable to grip straight bars with your upright rows in a close grip, it can cause shoulder impingement. Use a medium grip (shoulder-width), an EZ Curl bar, or a low pulley with a rope attachement to allow for greater freedom of movement.

Split squats will stretch your hip flexors. However if they are tight they can tear. To decrease the range of motion, do 90/90 splitsquats. If you have a high level of flexibility, elevate the front-foot onto a step.

The gym is seeing more distal biceps tear from preacher curls or heavy bent-knee Deadlifts. Avoid this by using a pronated grip in both exercises. To put it another way, don't use a mix grip on deadlifts. Use only a double, overhand grip.

Avoid performing deadlifts in mixed-grip grip to lessen your chance of injury.

(Photo by Victor Freitas

That was Once, This is Now

Some exercises go bad over time, not unlike fine wine. We've already discussed a few of them. You may have to use discretion in some cases, pardon the pun!

Although they may have worked for you when your were younger, now they hurt your knees. Instead, you can do stationary lunges (also known split squats), or step ups. If those are still a problem, you may be able to do single-leg leg work on a leg extension or leg press.

If skull crushers destroy your elbows, do pressdowns instead. If high-pulley pressdowns are too painful, you can do them with elastic resistance. Simply drape an elastic tube or band over your chin and give it a try.

Tendon ruptures don't come as a joke. I hate to say it, but they are more common with age. Be smart. Do not attempt a onearm chin-up while you are a teenager. Attempting it later in your life is a mistake. You can either stick to two-arm pulldowns or you can keep it that way if you feel too aggressive.

Nordic curls and glute ham raises were two exercises that worked well for you as a younger person, but are now too difficult on your hamstrings. Instead, stick with leg curls where you are better able to control the load.

Two Issues of Press

Most gym rats are "pushers," not "pullers." They do too much horizontal pushing and not enough vertical pushing. If 100-pound dumbbells are easily pressed flat on your stomach, then you should be in a position to push 70-pound dumbbells overhead. A great antagonist to the standing, one-arm dumbbell presses is the half-kneeling single-arm cable pulldown.

My book The Elite Trainer discusses how pressing force decreases between a down lying position and a sitting upright position. You are putting yourself at risk if your vertical and horizontal pressing power is not equal. You can also keep pushing forward if your preference is for rounded shoulders or a forward head.

Do Less to Get More

Strength training does not require you to run a marathon. Exercising for more than an hours is not only counterproductive but can also lead to injury. You can increase your volume by breaking up your workouts and not doing one long session. This gives you more opportunities to increase your anabolic levels and provides greater focus and energy. You will also be less likely to get injured.

Dr. Mike Israetel explains that you can either work harder or harder, but not both! Don't use too much intensity if it's not necessary.

Let's be clear: If you want your body to look more like a power athlete than a runner, don't train too hard!

Not Too Heavy

Bill Kazmaier, also known as Kaz, is one the greatest men to have graced this planet. Kaz, who is in his sixties now, said that lifting heavy weights has ceased to be a possibility as he ages. However, this doesn't necessarily mean you can't lift weights. Just don't do it too often.

It is risky to take a 1RM lift. Even a 3RM lift may be risky. You shouldn't lift anything heavier than a 5RM for multijoint movements such as deadlifts/squats, presses, presses, chin ups, and rows once you reach your thirties. A 8RM should be sufficient for single-joint movement, such flyes or lateral raises.

Newton's Second Law of Motion states that force is equal in magnitude to acceleration. If you are overweight, the force that it exerts on your body can be very strong. In addition, injury can result if your structure is compromised. When used with high acceleration and ballistic speed, a light weight can put a lot of force on the body.

As stated in The Gift of Injury: "You cannot be 'above' any weight no matter how light it is, and you will pay the price for not respecting that weight."

A bench press is a simple exercise that anyone can do in the gym. One rep they'll lower their bar to their mid chest. The next rep it will touch them lower chest. The next rep they'll touch their upper chest. Instead of doing ten reps each set, do ten sets with one different rep. To your nervous system, it's like doing ten different exercises. It is very unstable at the shoulder joint. This can cause injuries.

Christian Thibaudeau, strength coach says that "show me a man who cheats technique, I will show you one with joint problems."

Not Too Fast

The risk of injury is lower the more eccentrically strong a muscle is compared to its concentric strength. You can use eccentric training to protect your body and improve athletic performance.

This method of training typically involves multiple sets (6-6) of low repetitions (1-6) with supramaximal loads (105-75% 1RM). But, timing of the lowering is crucial. If you perform multiple reps, the weight should drop for 6-8 seconds. However, a single repetition can last up to 10 seconds.

You should stop the set if your speed of dropping below 6 seconds. It is dangerous and could result in injury. Charles Staley is a strength coach who says, "If I place 10 pounds on your feet, no problem." However, if I put a

10 pound weight on your feet, that's a big problem.

The #1 Gym Injury

The most common injuries in weight lifting are to the shoulders, knees, lower back and hips. However, the most common injury at the gym is from dropping weight on your foot. Don't allow it to happen!

A friend of mine had an injury that left him out of commission for quite some time. After finishing his squats, he tried to lift a 45-pound weight plate off the bar. The problem was that he had forgotten the 25-pound plates ahead of him. He quickly remembered the plate once it had crashed onto his foot. Imagine how awful that would feel!

One interview I remember powerlifter Dave Tate mentioning that of all the injuries that he had suffered throughout his career, the most painful was when he fell on his foot. The 45-pound plate fell on his foot, and that was the worst. Ouch!

Nick Tumminello, strength- and conditioning expert, shares a great tip. Make sure you place the plates so your lips face inward when you're benching or squatting. This will ensure you have a firm grip on the plates when you want to remove them. It will keep any "bombs" that might fall out of your hands from happening. You should also ensure your feet are sufficiently wide outside of the drop zone in order to prevent the plates from falling onto your feet.

A final piece of advice: Don't place dumbbells onto a weight bench. This is one thing I hate the most. It's dangerous for the upholstery, and it can cause accidents. Don't let this happen! You can either squat the dumbbells to the floor, or you can place them back on the rack.

Unloading the right way

Deadlifts, like all weight training exercises, come with risks. The danger is not gone. It is not uncommon for people to get hurt while unloading the bar.

There are two options. I've seen many contortions when using this technique, including holding the end of a bar with one arm and trying to lift the plate with the other. Standing outside of the bar, reaching forward and pulling the plate away, these are all examples of how it can be done. These are both incorrect ways to do it.

It is best to stand on the bar, with your feet facing forward. Grab the plate from both sides. You might need to step forward a few times to get the plate off the bar.

This is the correct way to unload a deadlift barbell.

(Photo by Victor Freitas

Stay focused on the task at hand

You might not know that your spine is governed by your eyes. Think about what it means if you go to the gym and a woman walks up while you're squatting and have a few hundred on your back. Can you see how you could get in trouble?

The trainee and spotter both need to be able to focus. While bench pressing, my right coracobrachialis was straining because one spotter was paying attention and the guy on another side was daydreaming.

A good spotter can help prevent injury.

(Photo by Nathan Dumlao

Flip the order

It is best to do the compound, multi-joint movements at the beginning of your workout, if you are still feeling fresh.

You can try isolation movements such as leg extensions and curls if you feel sore or achy in your knees. Leg extensions and curls are good ways to warm up your knee joints. Calf raises in which the emphasis is on the bottom (stretched), position will help you squat deeper afterward. My clients could only quarter squat and felt no pain. After some isolation work, however, they were able squat full-squat pain free!

The same logic applies for the upper body. Achy, sore elbows can be caused by many things. The most common reason for sore, achy elbows is excessive shoulder interior rotation. Doing some external rotate exercises first can help to fix this problem (more details in the next section).

Another reason is weak forearm muscles and extensors. These exercises can be used to kickstart a workout. If your elbows are bothering you, I bet it's not often. Forearm work should be performed first in your workout. Do more volume. It will improve your elbow condition and you might even end up with Popeye-like forearms.

Train the Weak Link

Injuries can result from performing the same exercises over and over again. Exercise variety is important. It is important to avoid repetitive patterns and injuries from overuse. You should even emphasize the moves you don't know. Remember that a chain will only be as strong or weak as the weakest link.

Focus on your weaknesses to improve your performance and reduce the likelihood of injury.

You can work on your weaknesses by training them first in a class. Prioritize the issue. It means performing remedial exercises and assistance before the main lifts. This can be done for anywhere from 8-12 weeks to more, depending on your needs. After you have returned to regular lifting, you will feel stronger and less pain.

The weak rotator, scapular and retractor muscles are two classic examples. If possible, isolate exercises for these muscles should be performed at the end or at the beginning of a workout. Stephane Cazeault (strength coach) suggests that these exercises be done first in your workout to close the strength gap.

Starting with weaker muscles allows you to prioritise them for greater strength improvements. In addition, the activation and warming up of the smaller stabilizer muscle groups will prepare the body for the primary movements which are performed later in a workout. Because you won't be using a lot of weight on these smaller muscles, cumulative fatigue won't hinder your progression to the big lifts.

You should also correct asymmetries. Thomas Kurz, author of Science of Sports Training says that injuries can be caused by differences in strength, endurance, or fatigability. This is also true if there is a strength imbalance of more than 10% between the same muscles on both sides of your body. This can increase injury risks by 70-90%. To prevent injuries, it is best to strengthen and extend weaker muscle groups.

Dr. Brad Schoenfeld, the author of Science and Development of Muscle Hypertrophy recommends you budget your work. So, do more for weak muscles or movements and less for strong. It's great advice.

The ShoulderHorn provides a great way to isolate the rotator and cuff muscles.

Beef up Lagging Muscles

Think back to any chronic injuries that you've suffered in the recent past. These likely happened in areas you are passionate about training. It is uncommon to sustain a long-term injury to body parts that are not well-trained or well-developed.

Change your habits if you want invincible. Let your "swole muscles" relax while you build up the ones that are slowing down. With a little bit of work, your body will be ready to fight for years in the gym.

Save Muscle Mass

Maintaining muscle mass is crucial as you age. Muscle mass acts as an insurance policy against injuries. It is best to use moderate rules in order to accomplish this task.

* moderately-heavy loads

* moderately high number of sets or reps

* Moderate tempos

* Take a moderate rest period

* Moderate frequency

It is also important to retain muscle mass for athletes of all ages, not just those who are lifting weights. A growing number of athletes are adopting moderate rules for in-season to keep their body weight down and protect themselves from injury. Think of muscle mass and armor. Keep it from rusting! Do everything you can for it to last.

Protect the Mafia's Strength

A cost is involved if you're an athlete looking for protection from injury. It requires hard work in the gym. Denmark research has shown that strength training is able to reduce sports injuries by 66% and overuse injuries almost by 50%.

There is a dose relationship between strength training (and sports injury prevention): the greater the intensity and training volume, the greater will be the prevention effect. In a Journal of Strength and Conditioning

Research article (Case et al., 2020), it was shown that injuries to athletes resulted in lower relative back squat power than in uninjured ones. In other words, athletes are less likely than others to injure their lower extremities if they can squat higher. Louie Simmons is a powerlifting guru who says, "Weak things can break!"

Although you don't want loading to increase too quickly in training, it is important to do so gradually and progressively. However, you have to work hard if you want to reap the benefits.

Al Vermeil knows more about training athletes than anyone. He is the only strength coach who has been awarded both world championship rings in the NFL and NBA. Vermeil states that athletes can get hurt the most if they push them to their limit. The best way to ensure that athletes get the results they desire is to train at a high level of intensity, but keep some in reserve. To train longevity, athletes and non-athletes alike, it's a good idea to "leave one or two reps in your tank".

Injury prevention means a significant increase in strength. This must be accompanied by a substantial amount of intensity and volume training. The old saying is, "The more you sweat in the training, the more you bleed in the battle." If you give your muscles that offer, you'll be well protected against injury.

The Core Problem

Today, there is much talk about the core and how programs should address stability and core strength. Let me ask you one question. What happens if your hand, foot or wrist is broken? While those are many questions, my point is to emphasize that the core must not be trained as an alternative to the extremities. They don't need to be mutually exclusive.

www.ingramcontent.com/pod-product-compliance
Lightning Source LLC
Chambersburg PA
CBHW041141110526
44590CB00027B/4086